Case Management:
Elevate, Educate, Empower

Editors:

Colleen Morley, President, CMSA Chicago (2019-2021)

Eric Bergman, Past President, CMSA Chicago (2019-2021)

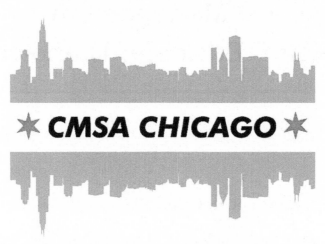

CMSA Chicago is a local chapter of the Case Management Society of America (CMSA). It is the premier professional organization, providing education, networking, and support to the entire case management community. CMSA Chicago brings everyone together to make navigating the health care system easier for the most important member of the health care team – the patient.

Published in the United States of America by CMSA Chicago
PO Box 7413 Westchester, IL 60154
www.cmsa-chicago.org
info@cmsa-chicago.org

Acknowledgements

We would not have been able to produce this compelling work without the tremendous support and efforts of the many volunteers who make our work possible.

To *Edna Heatherington*, thank you for the hours of editing and other support you have provided to help see the publication through for a third year in a row. Your patience and keen eye for detail have significantly improved the stories within these covers.

To the *many contributors* to this year's effort. Thank you for devoting your time to compose these stories, and for allowing us to publish them to the world. May these pages inspire you to continue sharing your stories to encourage and support the many beneficiaries, and practitioners of case management.

To *Deanna Cooper Gillingham* of the Case Management Institute (CMI), for allowing us to republish the winning and honorable mention essays of CMI's contest, "Case Management is…" We are grateful for the opportunity to give these remarkable authors an additional spotlight.

To the *CMSA Chicago Board of Directors* without your hours of volunteer work none of what CMSA Chicago has accomplished would have been possible.

To *Ellen Fink-Samnick*, a true friend to CMSA Chicago and a mentor to both of us. Thank you for once again supporting, encouraging, and contributing to our work. You are an inspiration, and we are thrilled to call you "friend."

Colleen & Eric

And finally, I would be remiss if I did not add a personal thanks to, Colleen Morley, *a true giant among case managers. You are an inspiration to me and everyone you touch. CMSA Chicago, and indeed our whole national organization, owe you more than we can express. Your enthusiasm, vision, and endless energy have enabled our chapter to far exceed even my most ambitious aspirations. You are an inspiring colleague, wonderful leader, and a terrific friend.*

Eric

A note from the editors:

While the stories in our anthology are drawn from direct and real experience, all of them have been edited to ensure the privacy of patients depicted in the them. All names and identifying details have been changed. Any resemblance to real individuals is purely coincidental.

Table of Contents

Our Own Stories

Foreword

We are at an important juncture in history. One year ago, when I was first approached to write this Foreword, nobody anticipated the year to come. The times have touched every member of our workforce in a unique way. I would be remiss if there was not acknowledgment of the massive loss of life and collective occupational trauma endured by society, and especially our health and behavioral health industry. However, at some point we must galvanize our strength and build for the future; *that time is now!*

CMSA Chicago's book, *Elevate, Educate, Empower: The 2021 Case Management Anthology,* will help reset your practice trajectory. The book represents the best of our case management workforce through storytelling and shared lessons. After all, every experience is for learning with inspirational stories advancing the knowledge base. Through this robust content, lessons are conveyed that elevate and empower every level of case manager, whether individuals new to healthcare's front lines or to case management, as well as those persons most seasoned.

Despite all obstacles, case managers, across each discipline and practice setting, heed CMSA's primary ethical obligation, to prioritize the needs of all patients and families of every cultural background. Daily challenges test each case manager's ability to assure the secondary ethical obligation is equally fulfilled: to engage in and maintain respectful relationships with colleagues and other industry stakeholders.

Ethics is at the core of every case management effort, providing a firm foundation to bolster every action. This past year has exemplified the durability of case management and our entire professional workforce. You will want to keep *Educate, Empower, Elevate: The 2021 Case Management Anthology* positioned within reach. When you sense your energy waning, this book will be your reminder of case management's inspirational and sustaining force.

Ellen Fink-Samnick MSW, ACSW, LCSW, CCM, CCTP, CMHIMP, DBH(s)

Reference: Case Management Society of America (CMSA) (2016). Standards of practice for professional case management: author

Introduction to the 2021 Edition

In the summer of 2018 Colleen Morley and I were invited by Anne Llewellyn to present as part of a writing workshop she had organized at the CMSA National Conference held here in Chicago. Colleen helped me organize an interactive session in which we encouraged and guided the participants to write a first draft of a story about case management. Those stories so exceeded our expectations that we realized we needed to find a forum for our peers to use their powerful narratives to promote our profession.

Colleen suggested that we publish an anthology. In less than 8 months, we – primarily Collen – brought the project to fruition with the publication of *Case Management, It's not Luck, It's Skill!!"* which debuted at the CMSA Chicago Annual Conference in April of 2019.

At that first workshop, we talked about the power of stories and how we can use them. Our thesis was, and continues to be, that Case Managers are the best situated professionals to serve to promote effective and sensible health care public policy changes. We coordinate the multidisciplinary health care teams, and see the issues from many vantage points. One important part of creating change is to increase the visibility and stature of case managers in the public arena. We can do this with our powerful stories.

In *A Call to Action: Reporting Data to Amplify Your Voice* the concluding article of Anne's *2021 Special Report: Stepping Up to Certification,* Anne Llewellyn and Kayoko 'Ky' Corbet, write about the importance of coordinating clear and easily understood data that demonstrates the value of the work of Case Managers, or as they called us "Helping Professionals." Among the several suggested strategies Anne and Ky recognize that "getting published by telling a story of how a 'helping professional' made a difference brings the theory of our work to real life experiences that stakeholders understand."

Colleen and I are working to do just that in this and the previous two editions of our case management anthology. By creating this book, we are working to popularize and demonstrate the important work of case managers. We hope these volumes will make their way into the mainstream and catch the attention of the public. We want them to be a vehicle for teaching new professionals, recruiting practitioners to the important work of case management, and to teach the public to "ask for a case manager[1]" when they or a loved one have a health crisis.

At the writing workshop in 2018, I told several stories to demonstrate the power and importance of telling our stories. I told the story of John, a client of mine who lived alone in Mexico and who I helped to support in my role as a telephonic case manager for a large insurance company that covers US expatriates with medical insurance[2].

As I told my story, I got so caught up in the telling that I made myself cry. Afterward, Anne Llewellyn asked me why the story had made me cry. I realized that I had failed to convey the full emotional impact of the story in that telling. That impact was still within me, and made me react to the memories of my work with John, but I had missed the mark a bit, since Anne, and others did not get the same emotional kick from it. That experience continues to encourage me to work harder as I craft my written

---

[1] In 2014 CMSA partnered with Angle Med Flight to produce a public service announcement about the work of case managers. It is a well done, 60 second spot encouraging the public to "Ask for a Case Manager." You can view it on the CMSA web site, http://cmsa.org, or on the organization's YouTube channel using this link: https://www.youtube.com/watch?v=2nJqsah5noU&t=58s

[2] You can find this story entitled *Alone in Mexico* in our first anthology from 2019, *Case Management: It's Not Luck, It's Skill.*

work, so that I can convey the full impact in my stories.

It is not an easy project, but practice and further experience have helped me to improve both my own writing and storytelling, as well as my editing skills. Colleen and I have worked hard with support from several editors as we have crafted our anthologies. The satisfaction of sharing those emotions with others drives me to continue working on telling my stories, and excites me at the prospect that our books allow others to enjoy that same experience.

Later in that same day at the workshop in 2018, after we had discussed the importance and power of stories, we set our group of attendees to writing a first draft of their own stories. After only 45 minutes, we asked if anyone had a story they cared to share with the group. Several of the attendees were brave enough to read what they had written. The power and emotion of those stories demonstrated that we were on to something special. Thus, the birth of this series of annual anthologies of case management stories.

Our hope is not only that you will enjoy and learn from the stores presented here, but you will share them with your friends, colleagues, families and clients. It is an important part of the work we will do together to, as Anne and Ky urge us in their *Call to Action,* demonstrate in understandable, simple, and compelling terms the value we bring to health care, and teach the public to "ask for a case manager" in times of health crisis.

Eric Bergman RN BA CCM

Memorable Patients

"Sometimes reality is too complex. Stories give it form." --Jean Luc Godard

Jeff

by Anne Albitre, LMSW

I met Jeff in the hospital. He told me he had been working his construction job when he had a sudden and intense pain in his abdomen. At the hospital he learned it was cancer. Jeff had a decent paying job and a home, but he could no longer work. He did not have a support system or family to help him. He needed aggressive treatment. I arranged to accept him into our new housing program for homeless people, since he was going to lose his apartment.

He started his treatment and I connected him to a colleague in our case management department who assisted him to file for expedited disability income. I took Jeff to the welfare office to apply for SNAP benefits. When he couldn't fit his old clothing due to weight loss, we went to the Salvation Army to get new clothes. I took him grocery shopping for his specific food needs and the Ensure protein shakes he needed to help maintain his weight and strength. We had 24/7 staff and Jeff built friendships with them and the other residents.

I started my journey as a case manager in a city in the Western US which has a large homeless and transient population. During my interview at a

Medical and Behavioral Clinic which also provides transitional housing for people with mental health and/or Substance Use Disorder (SUD) diagnoses, my soon-to-be supervisor gave me the rundown of the many barriers people face in obtaining basic services for behavioral health or SUD while being homeless. In addition to providing wrap-around services in their clinic, they also had several transitional housing locations for those who met criteria and were committed to an intensive outpatient program. I was interviewing for a targeted case management position to provide case management to clients in one of those houses. I would also spend part of each day at the clinic's crisis drop in center, where I would be completing needs assessments and starting the intake process for new housing clients.

During my interview, we discussed another problem the cities homeless population had and what the clinic was hoping to do about it. People who have cancer, or need outpatient wound care, physical and occupational therapy, or IV antibiotics, and are also homeless face barriers to obtaining outpatient follow up services once they leave the hospital. My soon-to-be supervisor told me they were partnering with one of the Reno Medical hospitals to provide short-term transitional housing to these patients who needed a safe place to go at discharge so they could continue their medical care. Patients can't get IV antibiotics at the shelter and it is certainly unlikely they will get to their oncology and chemotherapy appointments while living on the streets without basic needs being met.

So, I was hired to provide targeted case management services and asked to spearhead this contract with the hospital. The Directors and I created a mini-psychosocial assessment and processes and procedures for receiving referrals from the hospital, assessing the patients face to face in the hospital and coordinating their discharge into our housing. Once in our housing, I provided ongoing case management services until their hospital housing contract expired, that is, when their outpatient follow up care needs had been met (IV antibiotics completed, physical and occupational therapy completed, outpatient wound care clinic appointments completed, etc.). With each referral received, I would assess the patient, use my discretion along with feedback from Directors as needed to accept or decline a patient and coordinate their post-discharge plan. Process improvements and feedback were continuous throughout the first few months while I figured out what was and was not working while best meeting the needs of the patient. Most of these patients were in our housing for 30 days and would discharge back to the street once their outpatient needs were met. Some were connected to group homes or able to be reconnected with family. During the short time I had with these patients, we worked hard to address the socioeconomic issues to the best of our ability with the time we had. These are the types of innovative solutions that make me passionate about case management. Identifying a problem, brainstorming solutions, and implementing, assessing and driving change for better patient outcomes.

About 3 months into the contract with the hospital, I received that referral for Jeff. A few months after coming into our housing and starting treatment, Jeff declined and returned to the hospital where he was admitted for over a month. He called me while in the hospital and let me know he now had a permanent feeding tube and wanted to return to our housing if we would let him. Jeff said they taught him how to take care of all his feeding supplies himself and while he had the option to go to long term care or hospice, he felt at home in our housing surrounded by the staff and other residents and wished to return.

We agreed for him to return when medically stable and the hospital agreed to renew his housing contract with us. Jeff had lost a lot of weight and become very frail. Once he returned, it was only a few weeks until he called me into his room one day. He said he was ready to go back to the hospital. Jeff called me a few days after that from the hospital and we spoke for a few minutes. He thanked me for everything we had done for him and without saying so, we both knew it would be the last time we spoke.

There are so many reasons case managers do what they do. We all have that patient or story we look back to that keeps us going and motivates us and this is one of mine.

Helping "Jerry" Return Home

by Cassandra Wadlington

In my job at a major acute care hospital, I learned of a developmentally delayed patient with minor physical disabilities who had been abandoned by his family. He had been hospitalized for many months. Jerry was initially admitted for "seizures" in early February, 2020. I realized I needed to investigate and uncover the back story.

Upon speaking to the emergency contact/next of kin, a sister, I discovered that in fact Jerry wasn't abandoned. However, due to the sister not being a United States Citizen and her living situation with friends, she could not assume responsibility for her brother. She also informed me that Jerry was not a US Citizen; he was from a Caribbean Island where he still had family. The sister relayed that Jerry, her half-brother, was brought to the United States by their father. She happened to meet Jerry when visiting her father one day. Jerry had been living with their father and Jerry's step-mother until both parents passed away. Then Jerry was cared for by other family members until they too passed away.

I reviewed the chart and learned that Jerry was alert and oriented, and able to answer questions appropriately. I went to visit him and had a conversation, which showed me he had some developmental delay, but was appropriate and answered all of my questions fully. He was able to provide the name of his mother, father, and sisters, and said that he wanted to return to his island home and "all the good food." I contacted his sister to see if she would be returning soon and suggested that we might help make arrangements for him to return with her. She was hesitant, and then refused, saying she would be returning, but not soon.

Because there was no medical reason for his continued hospitalization, I contacted the island nation's consulate in the US for assistance. I was referred to the Consul General at the Embassy in Washington DC. The Consul took the call and confirmed Jerry's citizenship and agreed to assist with locating family on the island to accept and support him upon his repatriation.

After locating an elderly cousin who still lived there, we learned that Jerry's mother had also passed away and no other siblings could be located. The cousin was unable to care for him due to her age, physical disability and financial constraints. With this information, I understood that I needed to learn if there were any facilities that could care for Jerry on the island.

The only assisted living facilities there are for the elderly. There is nothing for the developmentally delayed. It was now September, Jerry was stable, ready for discharge, and asking to go back home because he liked it there. I continued working with the embassy as well as with his sister.

Then one day, I was informed by the embassy that there was a retired medical worker willing to care for Jerry on the island, and that the embassy was making arrangements for Jerry to go home. The only thing stalling his trip home was the COVID-19 pandemic, which had stopped all flights between the island and the US until October 1, 2020.

Due to his disability the decision was made that someone would have to accompany Jerry on the trip home. I was chosen for the task. While waiting for the day of departure, I had multiple visits with Jerry to keep him informed of what was happening and to ensure his comfort level with the discharge plan and with me as a traveling companion. We also kept his sister informed of Jerry's status and discharge plan.

Working with the embassy and the Minister of Health on the island, we coordinated Jerry's new residence and finalized the plans for who would provide care once he was repatriated. Jerry was provided with a donated ticket, clothing (purchased and donated by the staff at the hospital), a 6-month supply of medication, a wheelchair, and personal protective equipment.

On October 3, 2020 Jerry was discharged and I traveled with him. Upon clearing customs, Jerry was able to visit with his cousin who had been brought to the airport by friends, and was introduced to his new caregiver and the Minister of Health. The embassy had made the family arrangements once the arrival date was set. Jerry and his cousin recognized each other and both were smiling and hugging in the airport. The cousin was provided with the contact information for Jerry in his new living situation, prior to Jerry's departure to his new home.

Since the trip, I have inquired about Jerry, and learned through my contact at the embassy that he continues to do well.

Geriatric Care Manager;
One Family's Journey

by Louise (who wishes to remain anonymous)

We are a fairly typical story among my age group. My brothers, Douglas and Frederick and I, Louise, are all in our mid50's with family and job obligations where we live far from our parents who live in New Mexico. Our parents are in their late 80's and want to continue to live at home, but need more assistance with figuring out modern life than we can offer by phone and yearly trips.

About 5 years ago, we heard Visiting Angels advertise their services on NPR and tried using them to assist my father with remembering to take medications when my mother Ann traveled several times a year. He was at first quite resistant to having anyone check on him. As he became a bit less sure footed and his vision deteriorated, I insisted. I told him that even I don't go days without anyone seeing me. He finally agreed to the Visiting Angels services.

Three years ago, my father, Patrick came down with an infection (UTI) which also affected his cognition as it often does in the elderly. He was hospitalized for a number of days and I flew to my parents' house for a week to help out when he came home. It was clear that my mother was overwhelmed with the responsibilities of managing an increasingly needy husband while shopping, cooking, cleaning etc. She would not accept help other than more hours of Visiting Angels to help with breakfast, and bedtime routines, but adding some support to her days, helped her a lot.

When we saw our parents in January 2020, it was clear that Patrick was becoming much less steady on his feet, the house needed to be modified for better safety, and mom needed more help. None of us had an idea how to find a local person to guide us through this next phase, and our parents, who had always known just how everything should happen, were beginning to lean on us. My brothers and I began searching the internet for senior services (not useful in NM), for aging at home help (no resources) etc. One constant remained, Mom and Dad were adamant that they wanted to age at home.

A therapist friend sent a site to me that included several links to Albuquerque resources including Visiting Angels and others like them. We divided them up and began interviews over a period of weeks. The owner of one of the services said he had worked with a Geriatric Case Manager with good results and gave us her name. It turned out, she was also on the list. We were not familiar with the work, or even the existence of Geriatric Case Managers prior to this.

After interviewing two Geriatric Case Managers, we hired one (Susan) in July 2020 to work with us and our parents. She began interviews with them in August and I immediately felt a huge sense of relief. I was able to relax my worry that I would get a call on a random morning meaning I had to drop everything, because one of my parents had a medical (or dental, or car, or house...) crisis.

In September Patrick suffered another UTI that made him unable to get out of bed and he was taken to the hospital. He was then discharged into a rehab facility. From there he went back to the hospital, and then back to another rehab for a total of two months away from home.

It has been such a help to have a case manager to rely on to help us through this. She can tell us which rehab facilities make sense (are close to mom and have a good reputation). She attends doctor's appointments with Patrick, and reports back to us so we can make informed decisions - neither parent is entirely reliable about reporting such details. She keeps track of Patrick's schedule (Ann still keeps her own). Susan coordinates with visiting Angels, has contracted to have a company evaluate and modify the house for accessibility, has found a doctor that makes house calls and specializes in geriatric care, and perhaps most importantly, can find the correct person to speak to at the hospital or rehab facility to check on Dad's status when Mom is frustrated by the system.

It has been enormously helpful to have a local contact that knows the hospitals, rehab facilities, and NM resources to advise us and make calls. I cannot begin to describe how grateful my brothers and I are for the discovery and timely hiring of a Geriatic Case Manager.

Taking Control of Our Health and Health Care

by Eric Bergman RN CCM

I met Vivian (not her real name) after several visits to the ER that occurred in three months. These claims had triggered an alert in our system. I work as a telephonic case manager for an insurance company that manages a number of insurance plans. The contract I was working on when I met Vivian is an insurance program run by the US government for past employees of the Panama Canal. We monitor the claims data to find clients that could benefit from case management.

Vivian was a typical example. Serial visits to the emergency room suggests the client has a chronic issue that she is not managing well. It suggests that she could benefit from assistance to understand her illness and learn better ways of accessing health care than the emergency room. From the insurance company point of view, helping her to see her doctor regularly and recognize the signs and symptoms of an impending crisis in time to avoid an ER visit, saves the company money. From the client's perspective, learning how to manage her care better helps improve her life by: feeling better, lowering stress, and having better control of her life.

When I met Vivian, early in the COVID-19 pandemic, she was 99 years old, living independently in her own home, and managing her garden and household, although she relied on her son for help when she needed to drive. She told me that she had been suffering from tachycardia (a rapid heartbeat) which woke her up early in the morning on some days. Usually, it would resolve and she could feel better throughout her day, although she did not ever get back to sleep after an episode. However, recently the episodes had lasted for a long time which made her anxious and prompted her to go to the emergency room several times.

Vivian was not able or willing to go to an office visit with her cardiologist. The cardiologist was limiting all in person appointments to emergent issues, and Vivian's visits to the emergency room had resulted in normal test results and no diagnosis of a clear cardiac problem. She had been fitted with a Holter monitor – a vest that can be worn for 24 hours while it monitors the patient's heart – and the results of the test were not normal, but also not alarming. The cardiologist had agreed to "see" Vivian via teleconference, but because of Vivian's hearing loss, she had a hard time understanding and communicating with the cardiologist. Her son had been the one to do most of the talking and had to relay to Vivian what the doctor said. Fortunately, Vivian was able to hear and understand me over the phone, and this helped to increase the strength of our bond, and made Vivian willing to talk to me at length.

Since Vivian was not able to explain to me what the cardiologist had said, she agreed that I should talk with her son Rick (also not his real name). Rick told me several things about the visit with the cardiologist.

First, Rick was not impressed with the way the doctor had dismissed his mother's complaints saying, "Well, she's nearly 100, what does she expect? Her heart is getting old." Rick told me that most people who met his mother could not believe she was much older than 70. He pointed out that although she had a hearing loss, she had no other medical issues, except for the recent cardiac problem. She had never smoked and had no significant family history of illness. While he knew his mother was not going to live forever, she seemed to him to be a long way from death and had a full, happy, and independent life, which she wanted to continue to enjoy.

Second, the cardiologist had prescribed a medication for her (a beta blocker called metoprolol) which could help to regulate her heart beat. However, Vivian said the medication made her tired, and she didn't feel well when she took it, so she had stopped taking it.

Shortly after I had begun to work with Vivian, she had another episode and went to the emergency room again. When they still didn't find any clear cause for her issue, the ER doctor had convinced Vivian to take ¼ of the metoprolol pill each day. Now for those who are not familiar with metoprolol, it comes as a tiny pill. I was impressed that Rick and Vivian were able to divide it into quarters, let alone that it would have any real effect at that small a dose, but Vivian reported that she felt no side effects, other than the resolution of her tachycardia. Rick and I discussed that it might only be placebo, but if Vivian felt better, that was a good thing.

Unfortunately, after only a week or two, the early morning palpitations returned and Vivian was anxious. Thanks to her work with me, she didn't go to the emergency room this time, but instead planned another telehealth visit with the cardiologist. I had spent some time talking with Rick about ways to improve his communication with the cardiologist and helped him to feel more confident about pushing back against assumptions he preserved the doctor to make and to challenge the doctor to listen better to what Vivian was telling him. This time the cardiologist had suggested that she increase the dose of the metoprolol and that she consider an implantable heart monitor so they could get a better evaluation of her heart function. Vivian agreed to try the higher dose of the medication, but didn't want "anyone to cut me open to put something inside." The doctor had pushed her to allow a couple of weeks for her body to get used to the new higher dose of metoprolol, and Vivian had reluctantly agreed.

Not only had Vivian and I form a strong bond, but Rick and I had enjoyed our conversations. Rick, Vivian, and I talked about aging and living with chronic illnesses. One of my goals as a case manager is to empower my clients to take charge of their healthcare through understanding the details of their condition and the consequences of the various choices they can make. We had talked about end-of-life issues – considering Vivian's age it seemed prudent to help her think about her chronic heart condition in terms of what she wanted most out of whatever years she has remaining.

I am a fan of Atul Gawande. He is a surgeon who has spent many years examining our health care system and has written extensively about it. He has been a frequent contributor to the New Yorker and has published several books. In talking with Rick and Vivian we had discussed Dr. Gawande's book Being Mortal: Medicine and What Matters in the End in relation to our conversation about the ways our system does not help people live to the fullest, but instead focuses on keeping people safe at any cost and treating all illness to find a cure regardless of cost in time, money, or comfort. Dr. Gawande talks clearly and helpfully about evaluating the consequence of our choices. In Being Mortal, he uses a number of clear examples to discuss better ways to think and talk about how health care providers can better guide our patients to have fulfilling and satisfactory years at the end of life despite chronic conditions. This had struck a chord with Vivian and Rick who had been discussing the issue for several years, but had not run across Dr. Gawande's writing.

My sessions of case management are designed to last about 6 months, with regular check-ins to achieve certain goals. Frequently, my long term goal with a client is to help them improve their understanding of their condition and dialog with their care providers to become more effective advocates for themselves which will render case management unnecessary.

On our last visit, Vivian explained to me that she was feeling much better, having adjusted to the higher dose of metoprolol and had been having much fewer and less intense episodes of tachycardia. She explained to me that she had been thinking about her life and knew that things were going pretty well and as she wanted. She realized that one of her major fears about having an implanted monitor was that it might lead to some other complication that would ruin her independence and the life she was enjoying. She said that she understood the heart issue might be more serious and the monitor might find something that the doctor would be able to treat differently, but for now the medication was working and she didn't want to risk procedures or tests that might spoil that.

In my book, Vivian had fully achieved our long-term goal and I was happy to conclude our case management session with a conversation about our success. Vivian and Rick were both happy and left our session confirming that they will reach out in the future if Vivian's cardiac issues become more complicated or troublesome, but acknowledging that, at that point, they were pleased with the situation as it existed.

The Journey Continues

by Teri Dreher

My journey into the world of private guardianship for adults with disabilities was, in a way, circuitous. I never had the slightest inclination to become an attorney, and most of my personal experiences with the court had been frustrating, expensive, and had left me scratching my head about the justice system in general. What I failed to foresee, however was that when I started my first patient advocacy company in 2011, some of the clients we cared for over the years would eventually need guardianship. Attorneys would ask us to come in and help manage clients who had dementia, no POA, and dysfunctional families. Sometimes, we would need to care for people who lacked the life skills necessary to manage basic finances or handle their own affairs.

So in 2019 I started a nonprofit sister company, and hired additional specially trained staff to help us with clients who had complex medical comorbidities, as well as serious mental illness or cognitive impairment. I got busy reading and talking to every attorney I knew to hear their stories and what the courts required. I signed up for a course that would be required of us if we were to continue to work with wards of the court. (Not all of our clients need guardianship, but if they are "senior orphans" and competent to choose us to be their POA for Health, we will manage them long term.) I really never realized how complex and just how heartbreaking this work can be. As nurses, we sincerely care for our clients and patients, but it is difficult work, and not for the faint of heart.

Our first client came to us from a care manager working on a behavioral health unit. The patient was a middle aged woman with serious bipolar disease who had set herself on fire in front of her husband after an argument and talk of an impending divorce. This was her second serious suicide attempt in the past two years. Much of the house had burned down and her husband filed a restraining order preventing her from having any contact with either him or their two grown children. The hospital care manager had tried unsuccessfully to place the woman safely, but everyone refused to accept her due to the violent nature of her crime.

Once a beautiful woman with fine taste in clothing, jewelry and the finer things in life, her face was a ghastly mass of scars that extended over most of her left neck and shoulder and half of her chest when I met her. The skin grafts were fairly new and daily applications of creams were required for months. Her husband hired us to help with placement and general care management, and asked that we be appointed by the court as her legal guardian. She readily agreed.

We placed her in a supportive living facility for people under 65 and set up a beautiful apartment for her, bringing clothes and decor that were salvaged from her home. We worked to get her a wound care team, a primary care physician, and a psychiatrist who would manage her medications. The psychiatrist in the facility agreed to sign the CCP211 document the courts require that would certify that she was unable, due to mental illness, to manage any of her personal or financial affairs. We also got her into an intensive outpatient program a few miles away that she would attend daily, get individual and group counseling, and process her terrible grief over the losses that she had experienced. But, she quit the program after two days, because of an anxiety attack. She cried uncontrollably after hearing group members talk about their family issues, because she no longer had a family.

We cared for this sweet, intelligent, and sensitive woman for over a year. No medication protocols helped her. She isolated in her room most of every day, walking around like a zombie due to her high dose medicines, unable to understand why her family had abandoned her. We finally got her to smile a few times when taking her shopping or playing games with her, but mostly she just cried every time we saw her, silent with tears running down her scarred face.

Then one day, she sent her ex -husband a text asking for money, which he did not answer. Three hours later, she walked outside the facility, hailed a taxi and went to a famous local shopping mall, where she and her family had made many happy memories when her children were young. They had shopped and enjoyed special meals there. She took the glass elevator to the seventh floor and jumped to her death on the Mezzanine below.

She left no note, just her ID in her pocket which the police used to find her ex-husband and notify him a day later. We found out twenty-four hours after her death when she had missed three meals. The police confirmed our worst suspicions right before they notified her family. We were all shocked and heartbroken. It was really a big wake up call to us all that getting into the business of guardianship would be challenging. And it has been.

However, there is a huge societal need, so we persevere. Most of the time, it is very rewarding to be able to protect and do care management for people who simply have no one else to help. It is a mission, and a calling.

Fighting Irish

by Aishling Dalton-Kelly

Does case management happen in home care? You better believe it does! I would like to tell you how case management took place in a home care setting when the need was least expected.

Let me introduce you to Patrick, a devout Catholic born and raised in the midwest. Patrick required home care services when he was diagnosed at the early age of just 67 with the onset of dementia. Patrick was an only child who had no living relatives and Aishling companion home care took care of him for almost 8 years.

Fortunately for Patrick his mother had been an extremely strong, hardworking Irish Catholic woman who worked around the clock so that her only son could attend a Catholic high school and college. By the grace of God, at college he met his lifelong friends and future guardian angels, who in later years took care of Patrick like brothers - in essence they were his family. They and I called ourselves Team Patrick!

Patrick worked for the city and was well connected, known, loved, and respected everywhere he went. Everyone knew and adored him! He became a major recruiter and advocate for his Catholic high school, even during his dementia when he could not string a sentence together. On any given outing to a store, a walk around the block, or a social gathering, Patrick was drawn like a magnet to any adolescent boy, to recruit for his alma mater.

Many days the caregivers and I got into a bartering discussion as we tried to get him to wear a clean jacket outside instead of his old high school jacket that he preferred to wear. We could not get him to take it off. Often it badly needed washing, but we just let him wear it, because it was his beacon of strength. He was so proud to wear it, even in inclement weather. He was a massive sports fan and attended the school's every wrestling and football game during the years we took care of him.

It was during one of these games that a strange lady appeared and consistently sat herself close to Patrick. She appeared to be quite an educated woman and she worried us all, because she seemed to know so much about Patrick. My caregivers would report that this lady started to show up more and more at the games and encouraged and enticed him into conversations, conveniently making references to all the people he would have known during his years at school. Patrick was always a dashing, charming, and mannerly gentleman no matter who he spoke to, but this relationship concerned us all.

We were hired to take care of him 6 hours a day at first. We came in at noon Monday thru Friday and assisted him with activities of daily living and as time went on and his condition worsened, we moved to providing 24/7 care. Patrick had to give up driving, because of his progressing illness, and to replace the car we felt he needed a distraction. I suggested a dog. Patrick got his dog and we walked her daily. It became the highlight of Patrick's day to walk Rita proudly around his neighborhood.

After a few months of this lady conveniently showing up at the games, phone numbers were exchanged, and we noted that Patrick was having conversations with her when we were not there. Patrick had difficulty talking because of his illness, so she did most of the talking and then shouting when she would get frustrated that he could not respond appropriately. The caregivers reported to me.

A detailed plan of care had been put in place before Patrick met this lady. He put it in place himself, knowing his early diagnoses. He had assembled several attorneys, in addition to his school buddies, and his best friend's son, who was like Patrick's own son.

The caregivers began to report that the new lady friend was now coming over to the house. We noticed on one of his credit cards bills that money was being spent on Friday and Saturday evenings at restaurants and pizzerias. His financial power of attorney called me to ask why these expenses were being charged to his credit card. I had absolutely no idea.

It turned out that the lady friend was visiting Patrick in his home on the weekends when she knew we did not provide care. She would get him to take her out to dinner or to order in. The charges were made at four- and five-star restaurants in the city and included copious bottles of wine on the bills. It became a big concern for "Team Patrick" as time went on. My caregivers told me that when they would arrive for shift on Monday the lady's car was in his driveway; she was now sleeping over. It became clear that she was financially abusing Patrick, in addition to verbally abusing him. Over the course of six months they blew through thousands and thousands of dollars that Patrick needed for his own care.

"Team Patrick" came up with a plan and we organized an intervention. Patrick acknowledged everything we presented through a PowerPoint with photographs that we had put together to help demonstrate what was going on. I am still saddened when I reflect on how vulnerable, frail and shocked he was at what we showed him. I will never forget his expression when we told him, "This woman does not care about you. She just cares about your money. She's a predator, Patrick."

He agreed and thanked us for looking out for him and sadly left the intervention, but ten minutes later had no recollection of it ever occurring. We tried to encourage him and give him as much control in his own life as we could. We encouraged him daily to tell her she had to leave, but he was not able to do that.

With the help of his attorneys and the court system we obtained a restraining order. She violated the order multiple times. The situation spiraled out of control and the case became very tense for all involved. Eventually the woman was jailed temporarily for her behavior, admitted to a psych unit, and died a few months thereafter. In short, we had to become case management and take over this entire situation for his protection.

Many families think that home care is casual, but at least in this instance, I can demonstrate to you that it's complicated and involves multiple disciplines that aren't necessarily written on the care plan when starting out with new clients.

I was so proud to be able to work with such an amazing team of upstanding, principled, dedicated, and genuine individuals who at all times put the client first. My almost 8 year journey with Patrick and his dementia will forever hold a special place in my heart most especially two days before he passed under the care of hospice when I held his hand and whispered in his ear, "Patrick, 'Team Patrick' is always here for you, we love you." He ever so gently and weakly squeezed my hand. Even through his dementia, he knew his team was there for him to the very end. Thank you, Team Patrick, gone but never forgotten!

Meeting Clients Where They Are, Even When They are Far Away

by Jennifer Axelson, LCSW, CCM, CLP

You may have heard the saying "meet the client where they are". This implies that as case managers, we are to consider each client's individual situation, perspectives, goals, preferences, supports, fears, and anything else that could be an impactful factor on their stability, needs, and/or progress. It is also important to note that meeting a client where they are is not an approach only taken during initial interactions, but rather should be at the forefront of each and every interaction with your clients. It is only after you have truly assessed where the client is that you can develop a care management plan that can meet your client's acute and long-term needs while respecting their autonomy.

This can, however, be difficult when we are brought into a situation that has already devolved into crisis, we cannot evaluate the situation in person, and there are multiple factors at play that are impacting your client's stability and needs. As case managers, we are called upon to understand the situation, prioritize our interventions, collaborate with and coordinate services from multiple vendors, and calm a chaotic situation. This is when care managers are at their best and can truly shine. To illustrate such a situation, I will share with you the story of two of our clients, Bob and Carol.

Bob and Carol had been our clients for over 10 years. They both had multiple medical problems and they used Arosa, formerly Lifecare Innovations, Inc., to assist in obtaining second opinions, reviewing medical bills, and finding rehabilitation options. They had always partnered with us to ensure their stability, sought advice when issues arose, and then followed the advice provided. We helped them maintain their independence as they managed two cancer diagnoses, kidney failure, sleep apnea and more.

Bob and Carol loved to travel, and they never let their many medical problems prevent them from living the life they loved. During one of their many cross-country trips, Carol developed a case of pneumonia. Bob was worried and took her to the local hospital, 2,000 miles from home. While in the hospital, Carol fell and broke her hip and a simple three-day stay turned into a nightmare. Bob's health was extremely fragile and he required specialized equipment at night to manage his sleep apnea. He thought he could manage the situation and attempted to do so for a week. His daughter called us frantically, filled us in on the situation, and asked us to contact Bob to offer assistance.

The broken hip was quite problematic for Carol and she had appeared to lose her will to live. The hospital suggested a six week rehabilitation stay in a local faciliy, or a transition to hospice care. Meanwhile, Bob was staying in a hotel, was not using his sleep apnea equipment, and was getting more and more fragile as the saga unfolded. He began yelling at the hospital personnel and threatening them at every interaction. The hospital was at a loss and called in their patient advocate team. Carol refused to talk and was declining every day. Bob asked us to intervene and review the treatment plan with the doctor and the discharge plan with the hospital.

We found ourselves in a situation where both of our clients had acute needs and no family support present with them. The first thing we did was stabilize Bob and got him the needed sleep apnea equipment. Next we focused on the treatment of Carol. We all concluded that she needed to be home. This couple was overwhelmed with their travel nightmare. The hospital did not know how to deal with the angry, exhausted, sleep deprived husband who was irrational in his expectations. We all believed the best chance for dual stability was to return them home as soon as possible. A return home meant that Carol could rehab near her family and friends, and Bob could get rest and support.

We consulted with a personal injury attorney to determine if a suit should be filed for the broken hip. The family concluded that their goal was to get Carol home and not pursue fault in this case. This is where the family allowed us to negotiate with the hospital to get Bob and Carol home. We insisted that the hospital coordinate and pay for an air ambulance, fully staffed with a physician and nurse, to fly them home. The hospital agreed. Furthermore, we asked them to pay for transporting the car home so Bob could ride in the air ambulance with his wife. And finally, we asked for the hotel and all co-pays to be waived to which they also agreed.

The couple was transferred to a hospital in their hometown within three days of their call to us. Once she was in her hometown, Carol was able to focus on getting better. She completed her rehabilitation in a center one mile from their home. Bob was supported by family and friends, used his sleep apnea equipment, and visited Carol daily.

This was over two years ago. Carol was able to come home after her rehabilitation stay and the couple is living independently in their home. Carol is going to water exercise classes three days a week and is a social butterfly. After sufficient rehabilitation, she expressed a desire to drive again, which after significant testing and coordination, was granted.

This family needed to be home and together to recover from their ordeal. They are planning more trips this year, but before they go they are providing us the itinerary and will call us at the first sign of trouble, not after the fact. It is delightful to participate in improving the quality of life for these two people. We welcome the opportunity they provide us to help them face the challenges they encounter in the future.

This situation called upon us to calm a chaotic situation, for clients with different needs, all from thousands of miles away. Taking the time to meet Bob and Carol where they were, allowed us to accurately evaluate their needs, understand their perspectives, and develop a care management plan that successfully returned them to stability. This case has proved to us, we can still meet clients where they are...even if that happens to be thousands of miles away!

Providing Telephonic Case Management

by John Heraty LCSW CCM CPA

I'm starting my fifteenth year working as a telephonic clinical social worker for a large health insurance company. Since the beginning, I have had a front row seat in witnessing the undeniable benefits of telehealth to our members. The telehealth services I'm principally speaking of are the case management services provided by our nurses and social workers.

My story focuses on a member (I call them "P") who reported not being fluent in English and opting for our Language Line translation services.

A nurse case manager I work with frequently told me that P can seem combative, demanding, and verbose. I figured this would be a very challenging case due to language barriers and potential behavioral health issues. I was bracing myself for a tough call as I reviewed the case file, and researched the health insurance benefit plan and local community resources. I then did an initial outreach phone call with the assistance of our Language Line interpreter.

I was pleasantly surprised that P was receptive, pleasant, focused and had a healthy sense of urgency and intensity of feeling about addressing care plan needs. I have close friends and acquaintances whose primary language is the same as P's and I could feel a bond and rapport between us develop quickly.

P had a long list of issues and questions that needed to be addressed. This often required P, the interpreter, and me to make conference calls to various agencies and providers. P had been having issues related to diabetes which required special shoes. P didn't know how to get them covered by insurance. We discussed how P's physician needed to write an order for diabetic shoes with accompanying clinical notes and send the information to an in-network durable medical equipment (DME) provider. I provided a list of in-network DME stores near the house. P made plans to visit these DME stores to find the right diabetic shoes. Once found, P requested that the physician fax the DME provider the prescription and appropriate clinical documentation.

P also has recently had some specialist appointments and found that the copay charge was $5 more than expected. I coordinated a conference call to the provider's office and we left voice mail expressing P's concern and seeking clarification. Although I can't quote or confirm benefits as a social worker, I agreed with P that the copay amount charged was $5 more than the benefit guidance sheet. I told P I would follow up about the problem once I either spoke with the involved provider or our Member Services department.

Additionally, P had strong expectations that a bath chair was covered by Medicare, since they had been told that by someone at the hospital when discharged home. I again reminded P that I can't quote or confirm health insurance benefits, but I noted that a bath chair may not be covered by Medicare. I suggested P call Member Services to inquire about this benefit issue. I noted that Medicaid may possibly cover a bath chair. P expressed appreciation for my help.

I also consulted with P's home health care (HHC) nurse on a few occasions, prior to speaking with P, to ensure the home health care nursing needs were being met.

In addition to the health insurance benefit issues discussed above, P needed assistance coordinating non-health-insurance issues related to community-based and in-home services. This included getting access to the Office on Aging's in-home support services, and getting enrolled in Medicaid.

P told me they had left a message for the Office on Aging, but never got a return call. We did a conference call to the Office on Aging and explained P's situation and language preferences with the assistance of our interpreter. The Office on Aging representative expressed understanding, took down P's contact info and said she would make an urgent referral. She said that a case manager fluent in P's language would call to schedule an in-home assessment. P and I agreed that the assigned case manager could also call me in an effort to optimize P's care plan.

P also told me that they used to be Medicaid eligible, which would typically cover most of the medical expenses. P reported recently that they began to be charged for medical copays and other medical expenses. I explained how if P and their spouse are over the income threshold, they may be able to qualify for Medicaid via a spend-down program. I provided the Medicaid hotline number and explained that the representative there could screen for benefit eligibility over the phone. P also told me they have two adult children and I suggested they could help with this process. I also explained that the Office on Aging case manager, who speaks P's primary language, may be able to provide Medicaid eligibility advocacy.

Prior to my engagement with P using a language interpreter for case management, care plan agreement, and discussions, P had seemed frustrated by an inability to effectively manage the plan of care. P didn't have a good understanding of how to best access health insurance coverage, nor how to access needed community-based resources. With my support as a telephonic case manager, P was more relaxed and confident and progressively got the services needed at a cost that they found fair and reasonable.

P and I discussed how I would continue to work with them for as long as needed until they felt all of the social services needs were met. I explained that case management is part of the health insurance benefit.

This member experience emphasized to me the power of using an interpreter to optimize communication about care plan goals. I enjoyed working with this member and each of the interpreters that was assigned to work with us during our phone calls. These types of telehealth service engagements are why I got into the field of social work case management and why it brings me so much joy.

IMPACT

by Connie Sunderhaus RN-BC,CCM

Case Managers, Nurses and Social Workers do not just impact patient's lives - our patients often have a much greater impact on our lives. During some recent reflection on my career, many patients and situations came to mind. A few touched me in ways they will never know.

When I was a young nurse working in Home Health Care, we did everything required on our regular visits to our patients. There were no Home Health Aides or Physical Therapists on our teams. If patients needed bathing, we did it. If patients needed a level of therapy to improve muscle tone, we guided them in regular range-of-motion exercises.

One patient during that time holds a special place in my heart. She had recently turned 23, a trained classical pianist who had been living in New York City for her career. Things took a wrong turn for her as she learned she had severe Multiple Sclerosis. In fact, on her birthday, she came home to tell this horrible diagnosis to her new husband, and it was the same day the husband told her he wanted a divorce. She then moved back to Ohio to live with her parents, and it was during that time that I was assigned to her care as a Visiting Nurse.

She could no longer play the piano due to the physical changes to her hands. Walking was no longer an option and she was confined to a wheelchair. Her voice was soft due to the MS changes. We communicated and she shared that she was more disappointed by the actions of the husband than the changes caused by her disease. She and I were the same age.

Although I needed to maintain a professional relationship, I recall feeling the same rage as she did about how her life had changed. She has remained in my heart for years. I only hope that I had a small impact on bringing some positivity to our visits, which was one of my goals. Although I left the agency when I became pregnant, I later learned that her parents could no longer manage her care and she was transferred to a care facility. Some things hit close to home and impact our lives and practices as time goes on. She was my age, newly married as I was, yet our lives had traveled very different paths.

In later years as both a nurse and a Case Manager, I was chastised, even yelled at by physicians and patients. While these things were difficult to experience, I was secure in knowing I was following the appropriate procedure, based on sound principles.

For over twenty years I did occasional worker's compensation case management. On one occasion the patient's treating physician and I discussed with the patient the need for him to see a pain management specialist, as he was taking multiple medications for pain and wanted a way to discontinue them by finding other ways to decrease and manage his chronic pain. The patient was told the specialists would determine what refills were needed and prescribe anything going forward.

At the appointment with the specialist, I waited in reception while the patient had his private appointment. Very shortly after the examination began, the specialist came out to reception and chastised me, saying, "I don't know why he is here; he just wants me to refill his pain meds. This appointment was a waste of my time."

I listened, then asked if I could come into the room with both him and the patient. I was able to have the patient explain that he was told to bring all his medications with him and didn't really understand the role of the specialist. The patient said he did not want to continue taking so many pills. This gave the specialist a better understanding of the patient and an opportunity to explain his role in the patient's care.

This case impacted me by demonstrating the important role of the Case Manager as the bridge to improve communication and achieve the real goals of care. It happened that I was present and managing the care in that instance, but what happens when there is no case manager?

What could have occurred if I had not been there? Since he had a case manager, this young worker was able to transition off the pain medications more quickly, and I helped to prevent multiple, unnecessary physician appointments for him to achieve his goal. This was another instance where I felt impacted by this exchange and it helped make me a better Case Manager.

In more recent years in my role as a Case Manager consultant, I frequently deliver educational presentations for Case Management audiences. When receiving reviews, it helps me focus on the presentation – should it be modified? was my delivery satisfactory? etc. And it is nice to read those 'atta boy' notes that the program was considered very good.

However, the greatest impact comes from those audience members who stick around at the end to ask questions. Those are the ones that touch me the most. Not so much that I did my job, but that I connected with those individuals in a more personal way. There is no way to adequately describe that – other than to say, again my job touched me more than it touched the audience.

Many writers have tried to describe the impact we receive from our patients, colleagues, and audiences. All I can say is that I have been fortunate enough to have been touched beyond any expectation.

Making Concrete Improvements

by Amanda Bennett Williamson BSN, BA, RN, CCM

Case Management is the satisfying job of helping people live their best life possible by identifying their unmet healthcare needs and providing all available resources to help meet those needs by tying together the fragmented bits and pieces of health information patients are working with into a unified whole.

Per Deanna Cooper Gillingham's book, CCM Certification Made Easy, The American Case Management Association, or ACMA, defines case management as a collaborative process that assesses, plans, implements, coordinates, monitors, and evaluates the options and services required to meet the client's health and human services needs. It is characterized by advocacy, communication, and resource management and promotes quality and cost-effective interventions and outcomes (page 2).

That definition and those elements are important, but the real joy in case management, for me, comes in helping people, one individual at a time, achieve better health through finding out exactly what they need, what's keeping them from getting that, and helping them get integrated care to help them live their lives as freely and happily as possible. Individual patient stories demonstrate how these principles are put into action! As a telephonic case manager for an insurance company, I would like to share a member story that demonstrates some of these principles and actions.

One day, I called a member, we'll call her Michelle, who had poorly managed diabetes and had suffered a stroke which resulted in speech difficulties. Michelle lived alone, but her daughter was available to help her with her healthcare. Her daughter, we'll call her Amy, said "Mom wants to manage her diabetes better, and I know that checking her sugars is important, but with her fixed income she just cannot afford to buy a machine, never mind everything else, like those strips and the needles. I know diet is important, too, but it's just so hard to eat healthy food, and it's so expensive! And she really doesn't know what to eat. Plus, she can hardly talk right anymore. I've called her doctor a few times, and she's getting home health, but for some reason, they still haven't sent out a speech therapist. We just don't know what to do." Amy agreed to work with the Case Manager to find what her mother would need to best manage her conditions, but sounded doubtful that the case manager would be able to help. Sometimes, despite our best efforts as case managers, we are not able to help and that's disappointing. But I am always determined to do everything possible to help these members get the care they need.

Here are the action steps I took to get the member what she needed and was entitled to.

Planning: My plan included finding resources for Michelle to obtain diabetic testing supplies for free and arrange for this member to get home speech therapy. Also, we discussed some ways to improve her diet on that phone call, and Michelle and Amy were able to determine some simple changes that the member could start on right away, such as drinking Diet Coke instead of regular Coke, eating more vegetables, and substituting a light evening snack such as cheese and crackers, rather than pie or ice cream for dessert before bedtime. I also offered a Social Work Consult to address the issue of difficulty affording nutritious food, which she accepted. Michelle was able to take some concrete measures to improve her diabetic management right away, after just one phone call, and was referred to Social Services.

Luckily, in this case, success with obtaining diabetic supplies was quick. To facilitate the goal of getting the member a glucometer, strips, and lancets, I called this member's pharmacy and determined that she qualified to get free diabetic testing supplies. Resource management was achieved by providing needed diabetic supplies that were already covered by her insurance – she just didn't know how to access this. This was an easy and cost-effective solution to this problem.

Care coordination: Care coordination involved speaking with Michelle's physician's office to make sure the diabetic supply order was sent to the pharmacy in a timely manner, then following up with the pharmacy to make sure they had received the order.

Advocacy: I advocated for Michelle by being persistent with calling her MD office until home Speech Therapy was ordered and initiated.

One week later, Michelle had received her glucometer and had started Speech Therapy. Amy was still speaking on Michelle's behalf, due to Michelle's speech difficulty. I discussed Michelle's results with Amy, which were very encouraging, with her blood sugar levels averaging less than 120, whereas before, her levels were frequently approaching 200. Michelle had implemented some medicine adjustments and had improved her diet as well, and was really proud that her blood sugar results reflected that. Amy said, "It's just really nice to get some feedback about how all of this is working! And she hardly misses her Cokes at all! I haven't seen a whole lot of improvement in my mom's speech yet, but I can tell she's encouraged that a therapist is working with her, and I know it will get better. Plus, the social worker called, and we have filled out an application for food assistance. I hope Mom qualifies!" It made me so happy to hear the change in her voice, which was dull and discouraged on our first call, full of hope and optimism on our second call.

My Case Management efforts helped Michelle make concrete improvements in her health, and while they are not terribly dramatic, they will make a huge impact in her life, and that's one aspect of why Case Management is such satisfying work. There will be some dramatic cases, but most of them are more subtle – the patients that I help generally don't need emergency surgery right then, but they sure need help, guidance, and resources, which Case Managers are uniquely qualified to assist with. Helping one patient at a time, in both small and large ways, adds up to a career spent helping hundreds of people over time, and that is very satisfying indeed. I love this career!

Process Improvements

"Storytelling is the most powerful way to put ideas into the world today." --Robert McKee

The Case Management Process

by Jasmine Lucinda Alexis, RN, BSN, CCM

If you search, you will find there are many widely accepted definitions of what case management is. The Commission for Case Manager Certification (CCMC) defines case management as a "collaborative process that assesses, plans, implements, coordinates, monitors and evaluates the options and services required to meet the client's health and human service needs."(Certification, n.d.)

What is the Process of Case Management and Who is Involved in it?

The Case Management Process includes screening, assessing, stratifying risk, planning, implementing (care coordination), follow-up, transitioning (transitional care), communication post-transition, and evaluation. (Certification, n.d.).

The person involved in the case management process is the case manager. This is someone who establishes rapport with a patient and reviews key information related to the patient's health in order to identify whether or not he/she needs case management (screening). The case manager gathers information and identifies the patient's needs (assessing). Through the use of assessments, the case manager will assign the patient into one of three health risk categories (low, moderate, and high). This helps to determine the appropriate level of intervention needed (stratifying risk). Next, the case manager works with the patient to come up with an individualized care plan that addresses identified needs. The care plans include specific objectives and goals (short and long term plans) that are specific and measurable (planning). Then, the care plan comes to life. The case manager works closely with the patient, family members and medical professionals involved in the process (implementing aka care coordination). It is important that the case manager not only offers support but makes sure the care plan is on the right track (follow-up). Next, the case manager will prepare the patient and their support system for transition to the next level of care and ensure the continuity of care by communicating with the patient, their support system, and other members of the healthcare team (transitioning aka transitional care). In order to confirm that the patient has had a smooth transition to the next level of care, the case manager will reach out to the member to see how things are going and address any issues or concerns (communication post-transition). The case manager will assess the effectiveness of the care plan and its effect on the patient's condition (evaluation).

It is important to point out the case management process takes on a holistic approach and looks at all the parts that make up an individual (i.e. physical, emotional, psychosocial, and spiritual, etc.) as well as who makes up their support system. The process is not linear or cyclical. Some steps might be completed at the same time and also might be repeated until the desired outcome is achieved.

Why is Case Management Important?

I became a nurse because I wanted to help people and my work in the medical ICU allowed me many opportunities to make a difference in someone's life. But I always felt like something was missing. Once my patient was stable, they would transfer out of the ICU to the regular floor and 99% of the time, I would never know what happened to that patient. And I didn't like that I only got to see a part of the story. So, in 2018, I made the decision to transition to case management. At times, I do miss the bedside but becoming a case manager has been one of my best decisions because I see the vital and important role I play in the healthcare field.

Through my time as a nurse and case manager, I can see how difficult it can be for someone to navigate the healthcare system especially when you add complex health conditions and lack of social support to the mix. Oftentimes, individuals do not just need care in the healthcare system but also in the social service system, such as help with securing housing and/or food sources, transportation issues, ability to afford medication, etc. All of these obstacles play a critical role in the wellness of the person. All these obstacles can create a "non-compliant patient." If we take the time to find out the true root of the problem, we would find that a person is "non-compliant" for multiple reasons. And once we address those barriers, the patient can get the tools they need to succeed in managing their disease, which leads to better patient outcomes and better compliance.

I won't sit here and sell case management as a "fairy tale" because there are difficult cases with many obstacles, sometimes the patient being one. But even on my most challenging days, being a case manager has been extremely gratifying.

Work Cited: "Definition and Philosophy of Case Management." Definition and Philosophy of Case Management | Commission for Case Manager Certification (CCMC), ccmcertification.org/about-ccmc/about-case-management/definition-and-philosophy-case-management.

The Case Manager

by Carolyn G Dunbar MSN RN

The job of a case manager
To others is sometimes hard to describe,
Because we can take care of our clients
With dignity, without actually standing by their side.

Because in the healthcare field,
If you're not specifically hands-on,
Others may try to judge you
Because you're not physically tired and worn.

But case managers do get tired,
And there's proof that it's true,
Although sometimes it's very extensive
To explain what case managers do.

For some think case management is an easy job:
They think we only talk to clients on the phone
They don't understand we also go through trial and
tribulations
Trying to keep our clients healthy in their home.

You see case management is not new:
It's been around for over 90 years.
We've been toiling and managing for our clients
Sometimes through blood, sweat, and tears.

Case management was started for clients who had chronic
illnesses,
Whose care was looked over in a rush,
Not realizing that these clients need more guidance

And not just our special touch.
So a case manager goes the extra mile
To make sure that the supervision is there,
To ensure that the client gets the best treatment they
deserve,
And seamless transition to excellent health and care.

Now there are many different types of case managers
But they all fill a similar role:
To advocate for the client,
Because we all have the same goal.

Sometimes case managers are not liked,
And some think we are health-care bullies,
But we know the purpose of our job
And we put our heart into it fully.

Case managers have a code of Ethics,
And this is for a reason:
The case manager's scope of practice
Includes Autonomy, Justice, Veracity, Beneficence, and Non-
malfeasance.

So, case managers just want you to understand
That we are the client's voice,
And they put their trust in us
To make the right choice

It's not just the Client we take care of:
It's also the family that we serve.
Case managers provide precise and effective communication
So, both client and family can understand the treatment
they truly deserve.

Not everyone can be a case manager,
For not all have the assets by which case managers are
described:
Motivator, Coach, Educator, Therapist,
With endless Compassion and Patience on their side.
So when you come in contact with a case manager,
Just know they are trying to provide the best care.
To provide quality health care treatment for the client
Is a responsibility we all must share.

"You're Not Alone" ...Finding the Right Choices for In-Home Care After Discharge

by Linda Kuniki

The phone rings and a conversation commences with a family member who is distressed, not knowing what their loved one might need for care services in their home. What I have learned over the last 8 years as I take these calls is to remember what the caller needs most is empathy and education about appropriate services. It's common for me to say, "You're not alone, I'm here to guide you", this always seems to resonate with the caller as I hear their tone change. We all know that when we feel that someone cares we can be more relaxed.

However, in the age of Covid-19 those conversations have been different. Many families could not visit their loved one, so it made things more stressful. In addition, even though case managers or social workers connected with them they felt helpless since they couldn't see their loved one in person. They got more distressed as they were unable to describe what their loved one needed. Also, many people were being discharged needing both personal and skilled care, which requires conversation about both personal care and how to obtain and manage private-duty in-home care. The calls during Covid are also more emotional - we hear the tears as they talk. They must be assured that it is okay sometimes to not be okay... usually followed by saying again, "You're not alone, I'm here to guide you".

My goal for every call is to listen, educate, supply resources, and offer solutions in plain language.

The In-Home Care Options

During the calls I do some education, explaining that home care includes any professional support services that allow a person to live safely in their home. In-home care services can help someone who is aging and needs assistance to live independently; it is helping a special-needs child or adult; it is assisting anyone of any age managing chronic health issues; it is for recovering from a medical setback or surgery; or for those who have a disability. Professional caregivers such as nurses, aides, and therapists provide short-term or long-term care in the home, depending on a person's needs.

Home Health Services

Often, we hear about the doctor sending someone home with "Home Health". This is prescribed by the doctor with an order to an Insurance- or Medicare-certified home health agency that can provide intermittent skilled care, therapy or visiting nurse services. This is for a limited time, and may provide a nurse visit once a week, teaching and learning sessions to train family members on special care needs.

Palliative and Hospice Services

A hospice and palliative care provider works alongside an existing care structure and is not meant to take the place of a medical professional. Instead, the hospice care specialist will integrate themself into the care routine and provide pain and symptom management within any treatment. Hospice care is a type of palliative care which addresses the unique needs of people with terminal illness and their families. Both palliative and hospice care help patients living with a variety of medical conditions, such as cancer, heart disease, dementia, stroke, and many others.

Personal Care and Skilled In-Home Services

A licensed Private Duty Home Care may be a non-medical agency. These agencies can provide caregivers for companion or personal care. This is a service to assist people with their activities of daily living, which may include bathing, ambulation, meal prep, medication reminders, light housekeeping and more. These services can be combined with Home Health or the Palliative and Hospice Services to fill the gaps in the care with hours designed to help a family, even up to 24 hours, 7 days a week.

A licensed Private Duty Home Care may also offer skilled care services. These skilled care services are for nursing needs to complement Home Health insurance/Medicare. Private Duty Skilled services are an out-of-pocket expense. Typically, these in-home skilled services are needed when a patient is discharged with a ventilator, an ostomy/gastrostomy, feeding tube, catheter, or some other nurse-provided care. For skilled nursing services through an agency, it is required that an assessment is made prior to the need for services, in order to plan and arrange. After the in-depth skilled assessment, some paperwork is completed by a nurse that goes to the client's doctor. The doctor must send back approval of the plan of care (POC) and the orders for the skilled care requested. This process can take 3 to 7 business days depending on the doctor. If private-duty skilled care is needed upon discharge to home, arrangements need to be made about a week prior to the patient leaving a facility.

Private Duty Home Care agencies may be contracted with the Veteran's Administration, Worker's Compensation insurances, Long-Term Care insurance organizations and more. These are things I remind families to check, to find what options are available and whether they may be paid for by any of these sources.

Important Considerations when Choosing or Referring a Private Duty Home Care

> ➤ Has the agency received an accreditation, such as Joint Commission (aka JACHO)? Private-duty agencies are not required to get an accreditation. If they have one it was done voluntarily to verify they are holding themselves to a defined standard of providing care.

> ➤ Do they provide non-medical and skilled care? This is important should a patient need to have a more advanced care in the home. It's great to be with one agency that can do many levels of care.

➢ Does the agency provide a RN or a non-skilled staff member to conduct an initial assessment before the start of services? Do they follow up with reassessments at least every 90 days?

➢ Does the agency guarantee compatibility?

➢ Are the staff competencies tested by a nurse? This helps the agency know if they have staff with special skills such as caring for someone with Alzheimer's/Dementia, ALS, Parkinson's and more.

So Many Families and Stories

The agency I am with receives nearly a 1,000 calls a year and each one is a unique story and each patient is treated individually based on their needs. During the Covid-19 pandemic the cases became more complex.

One of Our Stories

One patient who had had a stem cell procedure needed ongoing infusions and personal care. One of the daughters was a nurse but had a family and job of her own so she assisted her dad when she could. Right from the start our Director of Nursing (D.O.N.) and I met with the daughters. Due to Covid our

D.O.N. went to meet their dad and do an assessment for skilled and personal care services. Because the infusions orders were constantly changing due to his medical needs, our D.O.N. visited often. He would have a hospital stay and we'd update and schedule for 24/7 care. When he contracted Covid-19 we called the family daily to check on him and them. He did not survive, due to Covid complicating his condition. One day near the December holidays one of the daughters showed up and gave each of us in the office a token of their gratitude. As with many of our clients this case hit us all emotionally as well. So, if you see a healthcare professional with a tear in their eye know it's because of their open hearts and dedication to serving people in a special, individual way.

Managing the Complex Issues

by Rose Wissiup, RN

What is case management? That is a loaded question that could entertain thousands of answers. It may be easier to discuss what case management is not but that is not what is going to happen in this essay. Case managers are involved in the critical aspects of the patient's care that does not involve a cardiac monitor or a Levophed drip. Case managers take care of the sticky situations that cannot be resolved with a PRN (as needed) medication or by repositioning the patient every two hours. A few components of case management include assessment of patients, assessment of families and caregivers, listening to patients, communication with fellow staff members, following and explaining Medicare guidelines, discharge planning, and changing a discharge plan on the day of discharge (just to name a few). All of these come down to one goal: The success of the patient. The success of the patient after hospitalization means something different for each patient. Each patient has a unique goal for the discharge plan. A successful discharge plan, in general, is one that allows the patient to be safe and healthy in their home environment, wherever that may be.

Advocacy, education, coordination of care, transition management, and cultural sensitivity are a few of the tools of case management. Using these tools and working with a multidisciplinary team are what help lead to the success of the patient at discharge. Having the right supports, having appropriate medical follow-up care, having medications, and understanding all of these items, are critical to the patient's discharge plan. Case managers are the staff that is looked to for working out the problems that hinder the discharge of a patient from a medical care setting.

Case managers, along with the physicians and nursing staff, help the diabetic patient to understand the importance of keeping appointments with their primary care physician and the dietician. When patients are educated on the importance of follow up, it will help maintain and improve the health of the patients. Case management educates the patient and family on what the home health agency can do to help in the transition between the hospital and the patient no longer requiring skilled interventions. The education provided by case managers is vital for patients and families to understand Medicare guidelines and the rights of Medicare recipients. Providing knowledge to the patient and caregiver empowers the individual to make appropriate decisions about health care.

Sometimes case managers advocate for a patient in a way that is not well accepted by others. As a case manager, I have advocated for my patient to make the decision that the patient wanted, but no one else wanted for the patient. The decision was for hospice. Case managers are the patient's voice in many instances, helping to explain to family and sometimes physicians, that the patient's wish is to not return to the hospital but to be comfortable at home. That patient's discharge success is to live life on their terms for however long that may be. The goal is for the patient to be safe and healthy in the home environment. Advocating for hospice can help the patient to meet that goal.

Case management, coordination of care, and transition of care just seem to go hand in hand. Case managers know the fax numbers by heart of the local nursing home and DME (medical equipment) companies. This is such an important piece of the case management pie. Ensuring medications or prescriptions are received, transportation is arranged, and the discharge summary is sent helps to ensure the continuity of care for the patient. This piece helps to assure the patient's health will continue to be watched, so that any adverse events can be managed with the least interruption of the patient's life.

Case management is now about following up with the patient after discharge to check on the success of the discharge plan. Calling the patient after discharge was not a standard of practice that I was taught as a new case manager, many years ago. It is now a routine part of the day to call the patient after discharge to see how the patient is doing at home. Case managers are involved in helping with situations that may arise a couple of days after discharge. People change their minds. Case managers are well versed in the knowledge that a patient may decide that home health care was the better idea for managing the IV antibiotic for six weeks, instead of outpatient visits. It may mean contacting the hospitalist because the prescription was not at the correct pharmacy. Case management continues to support and encourage an effective discharge plan even after discharge.

Google dictionary defines success as "the accomplishment of an aim or purpose." Case management's purpose is to provide direction and guidance for patients, families, and caregivers. The aim for case management should always be for the patients' goals to be met that return the patient to an optimal level of functioning. Case management is made up of many responsibilities, ideas, and skills. It would be near impossible to list all that "case management is." But case management is definitely compassion, knowledge, sprinkled with decision making to help patients' families have success in managing their health.

Making a Difference

by Terri Manayan, RN, CCM

Before I took a case management position, my experience was very limited while working on the floor of a small hospital. When I applied for a position with an insurance company, my eyes were completely opened to the endless possibilities of what case management is.

Truth be known, I really didn't even know the textbook definition of what case management was until I started studying for my certification. It is a wealth of knowledge, not only in nursing but education, resource management, planning, collaborating, healthcare rules and regulations, assessments, and more: case management is much more than a textbook definition.

Case management is wearing multiple hats, multi-tasking, and navigating our complex healthcare system to make sure we have investigated all avenues to ensure the quality and cost-effective outcomes for our patients. But case management is even more than that, it's empowering a patient to make better healthcare decisions, it's advocating for them when no one else will or they cannot do it for themselves, it's being there in the darkest times showing them the compassion they need and deserve, and being determined and resilient to find the resources to ensure a better quality of life. And sometimes we are the only voice they hear to get them through the day.

Case management is adapting quickly to our daily changing environment and navigating through uncertainty to ensure your patients are safe. It's staying on top of the latest knowledge and guidelines, working through barriers even in the most challenging circumstances. Case management is working as a team to facilitate the best possible outcome.

Case management is working with our growing healthcare population to achieve goals they never thought they could achieve and feeling the pride our patients show when they've reached a milestone in spite of the many obstacles they've faced.

But ultimately, case managers are the unsung heroes of our healthcare system who strive day in and day out to go above and beyond in good times and bad to get the job done. Case management is a job I wish I had gotten into long before I did but so thankful to be one now.

Case management is waking up each day knowing you can make a difference!

Ahoy Mate
Step Aboard for the Ride of Your Life

by Alissa M. Myatt, LCSW, CCM, ACM-SW

Case Management is...a treasure chest of riches or a map that enables us to better serve our patients and their families. I may bring my good intentions with the desire to aid a patient function at his or her optimal level, but it wasn't until I began studying for the CCM and ACMA exams that I recognized what a rich gift Case Management offers us to constantly grow and strengthen our skill sets. It gives me the tools to do my job well.

There are times as a dedicated practitioner it feels like being on a deserted island, like Tom Hanks in *Cast Away*. We must learn and be aware of the tools around us in order to survive.... think "Wilson" here. As I'm navigating the maze of complex patient care with multiple conflicting agendas at times, the Case Management Values help me remain grounded and focused on "patient-centered care." To: "not get swept up in the story but to stay focused on the symptoms and behaviors." I constantly dive into my Case Management Treasure Chest or pull out my map, confident that I will find the tools to do my job well.

Case Management also values communication and collaboration. That "show of support" and Interdisciplinary Team (IDT) work is invaluable to our profession. There's a proverb: "Go faster alone but further together" that resonates with me in our role as Case Managers and the "glue" we bring to the IDT where "connectedness" is the key that unlocks that treasure chest or gives us the ability to read the map more clearly, to better navigate challenges we experience in our daily work.

Nurse Case Management

by Jerri Medved RN, MSN, CCM

A question that a case manager often will be asked is "I thought you were a nurse, what is a case manager?" My explanation most often begins with, a nurse case manager (CM) is one of the most important nursing positions in the hospital for all age groups of patients. They are the glue of the care circle, in and out of the hospital. CMs protect, advocate, coordinate, collaborate from the smallest tasks to life-changing decisions. Bridges across gaps in healthcare are built, maintained and repositioned to the needs of their patients by case managers. Teamwork within the healthcare community to reach the common goal of a patient's well-being is often bound together by the CM efforts.

With the implementation of the Affordable Care Act, access to care has become a challenge, lack of providers in many communities creates long waits for appointments and decreased personalized service. During the pandemic, access was again transitioned to increases in technology-based healthcare, often problematic for the elderly. While navigating the changing medical community the elderly often fall through the cracks in healthcare.

Older people may be accustomed to personalized care where they do not have to advocate for their care, and may trust without question that what is needed will be done. Seniors often get frustrated and give up, angry with the amount of time and energy it takes to get an appointment, fight with an insurance company for a benefit they are entitled to, navigate the pharmaceutical community for affordable medications, and a whole list of other tasks needed for their care. This creates a feeling of not being important to the healthcare community. Case managers help empower patients and ensure that they are not alone as they navigate their medical needs. The patients that say "my daughter/son/granddaughter/grandson is a nurse," often have a better team to responsibly advocate, educate and coordinate for their family. My goal is for every senior to have a nurse case manager in their corner to be that person they can go to for help navigating the healthcare circle. To help the seniors in Michigan is one of my main reasons for starting a nursing case management company.

As primary medical care continues to transform, nursing has become a key component to the support, management, and success of caring for the elderly population. Case management is a path for nurses to use their knowledge base to treat the whole patient, often becoming the right hand to medical offices. With the increasing field of nursing entrepreneurs, more nurses are choosing to become independent of the large corporations that often limit the ability to manage cases by maintaining staff shortages and low nurse-to-patient ratios. Now is the time for nurses to step out of the safety zone and continue to grow the field of case management making a difference with senior medical care.

Many different studies have proven that utilization of nursing case managers not only improves outcomes, reduces healthcare spending, increases safety, but also improves quality of life. Patients, families, and caregivers express their gratitude for guidance. Owning a nurse case management company has allowed me to witness many positive results that leave a nurse feeling rewarded. Even if the interaction is just to check on the client by telephone, it is making a difference for the geriatric population. By showing compassion and being accountable to the client's concerns, we can gain a senior's trust and be effective in helping them obtain relief from physical, social and cognitive limitations and medical problems. Telephonic nurse case managers can reduce adverse drug events by reviewing and educating about medications, they can reduce unnecessary hospitalizations and ER visits, decrease healthcare spending and increase lifespan with guidance and support. Case managers' effectiveness can be seen across the communities.

I celebrate this week with my fellow case managers and thank you for being that special person that critically looks at the whole person and their needs. You are valued and a true asset to the field of nursing. Whether you work for a large or small hospital, insurance company, medical office, government agency or a small company like Care Resource Team, without you there are millions of people that would be lost and or forgotten by the healthcare system. Be proud and know you are appreciated for what you do.

The Gift I Waited for My Entire Career

by Sue Lopez BSN RN

My role as a Case Manager is relatively new. Therefore my experiences may not be what others feel. I understand this and appreciate learning more. I am still in the phase of learning from others and exposure to various situations.

What I feel Case Management is? That is such a question that it requires not one simple response. I feel Case Management to be a rewarding experience for those of us that thrive on the unknown every single day. No two days are alike. No two cases are alike. I am like a Gumby doll having to move my mind for many situations. Moving my responses based on their varied needs. How I approach most people is dependent on where they are coming from. I work with many that are not as knowledgeable, or don't have financial resources to be able to meet their needs for health care. Many are negligent of their own self-care and then become ill requiring the skill of their providers, nurses, other professionals, allied healthcare staff, and Case Manager. I may not be their direct RN but nonetheless, I am always an RN. As their Case Manager, I must call on my ability to relate to their social, psychological, emotional, and basic needs. I must try to find solutions for very basic issues that most people take for granted. There are so many obstacles in their paths and I work to pave the road for them, whether they can walk down that road, or must accept the changes they now have.

I feel with Case Management my ability to do assessments is put to the test. I must assess the person where they are at. I must ask the questions in a way they can understand. Then base my next question appropriately. How do I phrase my words? Am I watching my tone of voice? I can determine whether or not to explore various issues further. My gut instinct once again comes into question, as it always has throughout my nursing career. I listen to their responses with my ears and my gut. I am lucky I can read people quite well, so I am suited for this better than those that cannot. I am one of the rare Case Managers that truly loves doing assessments.

I feel that in Case Management I am doing the ultimate at patient teaching. I go with what is needed at the time. They may not directly ask the question but my ability to see things in the "big picture" helps. I must gauge when they are getting overwhelmed and do it in sections. This is also my favorite part of Case Management. Patient teaching is so valuable to each individual patient and their family. Whether I am teaching them about their new medication, a diagnosis, dietary guidelines, or helping them determine how they can respond to their provider, I am always teaching. Many current patients tell me "I always like to ask you because you explain it in a simple way I can understand." That makes my day! That is what I want for them.

I feel that with Case Management we are also problem solvers. We must piece together the puzzle of many issues. Why their MRI did not get authorized, why their provider selection of a certain medication was not approved, or why the request for Home Health nursing was denied. Or were they discharged to home yet we can see they need Home Health assistance from our assessment of them? We must coordinate their care for so many issues. What if they are getting evicted and they cannot take their precious dog with them to the shelter? Searching for safe places to keep their pup can be very daunting but so meaningful to the patient. How to help them when they feel their physician or other provider does not listen to them? Do we intervene or do we suggest another provider? At what point do we suggest they obtain some behavioral health work? That is handled individually based on many variables. Do we get involved and make their appointments for them? Or do we commend them when they can do this on their own? Once again, it is based on the individual and their background story.

I feel that as a Case Manager we must contort that Gumby body to respond to our patients. Do I present as the nurturing motherly type? Am I the direct, authoritative nurse with a no-nonsense stance? Or am I that kind open-minded listener? The kind that nothing they tell me will affect me to react surprised? Do I suggest possible solutions or just let them vent to me? Regardless of how I respond to them, this takes a skill that many nurses and social workers possess. Some of us truly enjoy the challenge with a difficult patient or issue to work with these people that need our help. The one skill I am still working on is how to react when a patient I have been working with for some time is nearing the end of their terminal illness. This one is not one I expected to feel so deeply. I feel the grief, their loneliness but also the peace and acceptance they now have. I must remind myself they were so appreciative of my role in their life. I must also nurture myself at this time.

I truly feel Case Management is the gift I waited for my entire nursing career. I worked so many specialties over several decades. I covered all my bases to be a well-versed RN. I didn't realize I was preparing myself for this position from the very start. My former coworkers are not at all surprised by my present position because of all the reasons I have mentioned above. It may have been a change of scenery for me to become a Case Manager but once I learned the technical aspects, it all fell into place. This is me; this is where I belong.

Meeting a Hiker

by Susannah Marshall, BSN, RN-BC, CCM

Case Management is...meeting a hiker on a mountain in the wilderness who has a sprained ankle, no flashlight, and is running out of water – and figuring out how to best get them back to safety using the skills and resources they already have — while also assessing the situation and finding additional supports and services needed.

A Case Manager (or "Hiker Support Specialist" (HSS)) surveys the land and looks and prepares for obstacles before offering to help (reviews medical records and utilization history, speaks with providers, etc).

The Case Manager/HSS then approaches the hiker and asks them how they are doing, if they need help, and asks them where they are trying to get to (compassionate care, motivational interviewing, goal setting, and rapport building by exploring the patient's needs). The hiker explains that they are staying with their uncle and cousins at a campsite 2 miles away, and they just need to get back to them (establishing goals needed for the treatment plan).

The Case Manager/HSS and hiker look at the map together, and map out the path the hiker needs to take to get back to the campsite (collaborative care, exploring and assessing the patient's needs, etc). The Case Manager/HSS asks the hiker to mentally trace their steps – have they hiked this path before? Have they had this kind of obstacle before? How did they resolve it the last time something like this happened (strengths-based approach to problem-solving, drawing on the patient's already established skills and inner wisdom)?

The Case Manager/HSS then asks if it is ok for them to look at the hiker's ankle (consent to care). The CM/HSS assesses the ankle, sees if they can put weight on it and if they are able to be mobile with or without support (patient assessment of ADLs, building care plan). The CM/HSS also determines if they are in too much pain that something more serious than a sprain has occurred, and explores the possibility of needing emergency rescue/airlift (further assessment, escalation of concerns to appropriate providers). The hiker and CM/HSS determine that limited weight can be placed on the ankle with supportive care/someone to walk with (CMs do not ask patients to do more than they are capable of doing, but encourage them to do as much as they possibly can under their current circumstances).

The CM/HSS asks to see what the hiker has packed for his hike by exploring their backpack. The CM/HSS notices that the hiker has a compass, water filtration system, cell phone, and a flare gun. The hiker states that they had forgotten that their dad had packed an emergency cell phone and that since they were only 2 miles away from the campsite, may have limited cell service they can use to call them and ask for them to come pick them up in their truck (utilizing current resources before adding new resources, problem-solving, exploring additional resources and social determinants of health). When the uncle arrives to pick the hiker up, the hiker uses their uncle for support to get to the truck (following treatment plan to do supportive movement only).

The CM/HSS stays with them, watching the hiker move slowly, monitoring progress as they start to put a bit of weight on their ankle, and adjusting support as needed (monitoring and revising care plan). As the hiker gets into the truck, the CM/HSS asks the uncle if he feels confident getting him back to the campsite and getting him additional medical support as needed. The CM/HSS confirms that the uncle has enough gas in the car, a working cell phone, and emergency numbers as needed (exploring potential barriers to care, safety planning, advocacy). The CM/HSS wishes them all the best and continues hiking until they meet another hiker that may need support. Rinse/lather/repeat.

I believe the most important thing a Case Manager can do for a patient/hiker is to empower them to meet their own needs as much as they are capable, and then to advocate for them the rest of the way. It is so important that we not overwhelm or push them beyond their current limits, as this can be disempowering, and potentially cause harm or be traumatizing. Sometimes this requires doing a little extra work for them (calling clinics on their behalf to get an appointment made, conference-calling with them to their provider office or pharmacist to get the medications they need) until they are stabilized – which is the advocacy part. The trick is finding that sweet spot between ease, challenge, and overwhelm. If we build a treatment plan around the skills they already have, and use approaches that they themselves have stated have worked for them in the past, we build that sense of empowerment and confidence within them that promotes healing and sustainable growth (hopefully beyond the time we are providing CM support so that we are not creating a false sense of dependency). When we advocate for our patients, this also role-models what advocacy looks like to patients who may have never had anyone advocate for them before, or do not understand how to best advocate for themselves. It also shows them that they are worth fighting for so that they feel confident doing this for themselves the next time they need to ask for help or support.

In addition to empowerment and advocacy, it is the Case Manager's job to always keep their eye on health equity using a trauma-informed care lens. What if this hiker had been lost in the woods when they were a child? What if their mother had died in a mountaineering accident? What if the hiker was 2 miles away from his uncle for a reason unexplored (did he feel safe around his uncle, etc.)? These are all things that as case managers we get to assess from a birds-eye view, with a holistic approach. We get to investigate while being compassionate. We get to think outside the box while being systematic (following trauma-informed care recommendations). We get to ask important questions, and we get to problem-solve. Case management is taking a 360 view of a patient's healthcare and social needs, figuring out what the barriers to care are, exploring if there are any additional hidden barriers to care, empowering them to build off of their established strengths to launch them back into health (or as close to it as they can get), and then advocating our butts off for them the rest of the way. Case management is an awesome job!

The Tools to Fix the Problems

by Jennifer Zentner

What is case management...if we are honest with ourselves, the answer changes depending on the day. Case management is advocacy, empowerment, facilitating autonomy, and assisting people in attaining their goals whether medically or personally. Case management can be a whirlwind of excitement, frustration, fulfillment, and reward all in the same day. A colleague of mine frequently describes case management as the junk drawer of the care team because "everything gets dumped on the case manager." When I think of a junk drawer, I think of the half pack of birthday candles, the random assortment of batteries that never seem to be the type I need, the pen that doesn't work, and the random thumbtack I don't need. I think of a drawer of useless possessions that don't have a place anywhere else. I don't think of case management as the junk drawer; I prefer to think of case management as the toolbox.

A toolbox is often stuffed full of random items, much like a junk drawer, but in the case of the toolbox, each item has a specific purpose. A well-organized toolbox is essential for resolving issues. Having the tool you need improves efficiency, increases productivity, and lowers frustration. A toolbox is put together with intention, each tool playing a part in fixing a problem. Sure, sometimes after a complicated job, the tools get thrown back in and don't look as pretty, but everything still has a useful purpose. As case managers with the toolbox, we are prepared for anything because on any given day, anything can happen. From suicidal individuals to sudden homelessness, we must adapt our tools to meet diverse needs.

Have you ever seen someone that fixes things for a living? Have you been in their workshop? Every tool has a home, every machine is well kept, and they can make seamless movements from one tool to another based on the need. An effective case manager has a strong organizational system and has all of their resources at their fingertips. We are responsible not only for managing whatever administrative requirements are placed on us given the field in which we work, but we are also responsible for lives. Lives that are at risk due to barriers to health, barriers to work, and often barriers to safety.

A case manager may often feel that they are being "dumped on," but in actuality, they are being recognized as the essential person for the task at hand. Some days are harder than others. Some days our toolbox feels empty and filled with inadequate tools, but the beauty of case management is that those days are balanced with days where our tools are able to help fix barriers and make progress. Case management requires flexibility, resilience, patience, tenacity, and sometimes a nice margarita.

Case management looks different depending on the field or position in which the case manager works. Years ago, I was a case manager for adults with developmental disabilities. In that position, advocacy was 99% of my job. I advocated for their human rights. I advocated for their wants and needs. And in one instance, I advocated for appropriate legal counsel. In that situation, I had a 22-year-old young man with the cognitive capabilities of an 8-year-old who stood accused of a crime he did not even know about. He was arrested, questioned without a lawyer, and as a product of the foster system, had no family support to assist him. With no law degree, I had to open my toolbox and reflect on what I could do in order to assist this young man. With the support of my supervisor, we created a fundraiser to raise money for him to hire a new lawyer that could advocate for him in a way that I could not. It would be easy to think of the added responsibility as "one more thing added to the junk drawer," but I chose to see it as a chance to learn another facet of advocacy. One more tool in my toolbox with the added bonus of helping someone in need. Sometimes case management is knowing that we are not the appropriate ones to meet their needs at that moment and facilitating the appropriate transition. This experience taught me that effective case management is balanced.

Case Management is a field where balance is key. When a case manager is able to effectively attain a work/life balance they are better able to think clearly and develop creative plans to help others. On a regular basis, I have individuals tell me "you are my angel" or "you saved my life." Those are the moments when I know I am not a junk drawer; those moments remind me that case management is essential. These moments help provide balance to the moments when my toolbox is empty and I have used all of my tools with no success. Case managers must understand that we can't fix everything.

In case management, the only constant is change. Change in expectations, change in work level, change in resources, just CHANGE. Case management is flexible. In every case management position, I have worked across different fields, being flexible wasn't just a good idea, it was necessary. On any given day we may be asked to change the assessment we are using, the process we use, or the way we document something. COVID-19 has required more flexibility than ever before. But we are flexible with a purpose; as a case manager, we understand that our flexibility allows us to continue to provide the individuals the assistance they need no matter what changes we are being asked to make.

To me, thinking of case management as the junk drawer just doesn't fit. The junk drawer has such a negative connotation. We are not junk. Sure, we are pulled in a lot of directions, and some days it may feel like things are just thrown on us continually. But if case management was the junk drawer we wouldn't be given the opportunity to step up and meet the need. As case managers, we are optimistic and enthusiastic. We are the toolbox, the essential backbone of the care team. We use our tools of being organized, resourceful, flexible, creative, resilient, patient, tenacious, and balanced. We take on the tasks that no one else wants because we know they are essential and life-changing. The next time you start feeling like the junk drawer, remember—nothing about you is junk. Case management is definitely the toolbox.

What is Case Management?

by Angela Gottschalk, BSN, RN, CCM

I have tried to answer this question many times over the span of my career. Due to the ever-changing healthcare environment in which we live, the answer seems to get more complex every year. How can something so complex with so many moving pieces be explained? If you are a leader in a case management department and interviewing candidates for a case management position, how do you explain what case management is without scaring people away? I am the Director of Case Management in an acute care hospital setting with close to 10 years of experience, and I still have trouble answering this question.

Let me start by explaining what case management is not. Case management is not always a Monday through Friday job. The hours are not always 8 am-4:30 pm. Depending on the organization the case manager chooses to work for, an acute care hospital, for example, they may be required to work on weekends and holidays. And if you are a leader in your department, you may even get a phone call for guidance on cases after hours. Case managers are not only nurses; they are social workers, therapists, or other licensed personnel. But wait, there's more!

Time for the good stuff. Case Management is advocating for a patient when they are most vulnerable and cannot advocate for themselves. It is calling the local sheriff's office to fingerprint a John Doe trauma patient with hopes of being able to identify the patient so their loved ones are able to be notified. Case Management is helping a patient and their caregiver understand how to better manage their illness by providing education and connecting them to resources in their community. It is knowing you can spend an extra ten minutes talking to your patient who may be lonely because some of the things on your to-do list can wait until tomorrow. Case management is taking a few extra minutes to help your patient use the bedside phone to call their family because they keep forgetting to press "9" before dialing the number. It is honoring the patient's right to refuse the most perfect discharge plan, even though they were agreeable to it two hours ago and you worked really hard on it. Case Management is listening with your ears and assessing with your eyes. It is knowing when to recognize when something is not right and taking the time to dig a little deeper until you get to the root of the problem. Case Management is giving patients and their caregivers the tools they need to maintain or improve their health so they may manage their health in the outpatient setting rather than coming to the emergency room and waiting for hours.

Case Management is knowing how to communicate effectively. It is recognizing complex discharges with barriers. It is coordinating meetings, better sooner than later, for the family and the treatment team to sit down together to discuss goals of care and options. Case management is having difficult conversations, happy conversations, celebratory conversations, and tearful conversations. It is communicating risks and benefits of adherence to a recommended treatment plan truthfully while still being compassionate and empathetic all while recognizing the patient's right to self-determination.

Case Management is knowing how to collaborate with others on the treatment team. It is helping physicians transition patients to the lowest level of care that safely meets their patient's needs. It is helping the treatment team be good stewards of healthcare dollars spent. Case Management is helping providers prevent duplication of services, diagnostics, and treatments. It is knowing how to become partners in healthcare and being able to build valuable relationships with post-acute providers in the community. Case Management is often not revenue generating, but it is revenue saving when done effectively. It is knowing when to use your voice and knowing when to observe and listen.

Lastly, Case Management is continuing education and never-ending opportunity for professional growth. It is being innovative and thinking "outside the box". It is not being afraid to share a crazy idea that may improve a patient outcome, because a case manager knows something great might grow from that seed. Case Management is an important part of patient care and patient outcomes. It is rewarding in so many ways. Case Management is here to stay, and I am honored to be a part of it.

As Different as Snow Flakes

by Jared D. Johnson, MSW, LMSW, CCM

When people first hear the words "Case Management," they generally think of discharge planning. However, case management is more in-depth and involved than just discharge planning. There are multiple layers to case management that include utilization review, utilization management, connecting resources for patients, and patient education. At the same time, they move through the levels of care, and of course, advocating for a patient to ensure they are transiting through the levels of care with the best outcomes possible. Honestly, the previously mentioned items are just touching the basics of what case management is.

Being a case manager is more than just following a clear set of guidelines while working with patients. Short et al. (2019) explained an increase in medical services and social and welfare services are becoming more apparent for the general population. Just like every snowflake is different, every person is also different. Some patients may require more extensive planning, guidance, and education while navigating through various levels of care. There has been more reliance from the general population on healthcare facilities for more than just medical needs in recent years. Patients are presenting with chronic illnesses. Some of these illnesses are being exacerbated by social issues, such as lack of resources, lack of education regarding the disease process, lack of a support system being in place, and the list goes on from there.

Additionally, multiple healthcare entities are either currently forming or have formed contractual agreements with other healthcare entities to ensure they are all making a profit to keep their doors open to serve the patients' ever-growing needs. While this is good for business, this leads to confusion for patients. Patients are not understanding the role of each healthcare setting they are currently being treated at. For example, a patient who needs long-term acute care (LTAC) would likely benefit more from an LTAC hospital, versus an acute care hospital. This example shows where case management proves to be not only beneficial but essential for patients to have the best outcomes possible.

Case managers can be seen as both the "good and bad cop" from a patient's perspective, depending on the situation. The good cop, if case managers can connect a patient with great resources, leading to the best outcomes. Additionally, for a case manager to be seen as a "good cop," the patient is generally also satisfied with the results. Sadly, this could also lead to a case manager being seen as a "bad cop" if the patient disagrees with the presented options on the flip side. Such as a case, where an individual underwent a traumatic injury and they do not identify as being "ready" for the next level of care, which could include skilled nursing facilities, home with home health therapy, etc. During times such as these, case managers are also tasked with explaining to the patients the risks of staying in an acute care setting, risks which could include, but are not limited to, hospital-acquired infections and insurance companies rejecting a bill for services rendered at the current level of care. Additionally, case managers could serve as a contact person for a patient's loved ones when they are not sure what to expect next in a disease process.

While case management can seem like much work, it is also one of the most rewarding careers a person can choose to go into if they have the heart for it. Just like any other helping profession, it is not possible to train someone to care. However, if someone does have a "calling" for case management, it is a career you can hang your hat upon, feeling like you have made a difference in someone's life. Not only with clients, the agencies that a case manager is employed with will also turn to the case manager to be the subject expert in multiple areas. This leads to the need to have multiple disciplines working in the role of a case manager. Each discipline will view a problem a patient or client is having with a different set of eyes. Nursing backgrounds will be able to understand better the clinical aspect of the needs of a patient. In contrast, a social work background will allow for the social needs to be met for a patient, such as a lack of resources contributing to a patient failing to follow a treatment plan.

References: Short, M., Trembath, K. S., Duncombe, R., Whitaker, L., & Wiman, G. (2019). Contemporizing teaching case management: mapping the tensions. Social Work Education, 38(2), 212–226. https://doi.org/10.1080/02615479.2018.1506428

You Know You're a Case Manager if...

by Ethel Walton RN BSN CCM

Case managers:

> ➤ introduce themselves to a client and the response is "so what can you do for me?"

> ➤ manage family demands like, "my Mom walked in here and she's not leaving until she can walk out." Even if the crisis has debilitated her and she needs rehab.

> ➤ have to explain why patients cannot just stay in the hospital until they are ready to go home, instead of moving to rehab or skilled nursing facilities?

> ➤ are the ones that have to manage the laundry lists: "I need a walker, the one with the seat and basket, a wheelchair, a nebulizer machine, home oxygen and a caretaker around the clock. Also I need an ambulance ride home."

> ➤ have to figure out how to make time for the client who feels, "I have to research all the skilled nursing facility choices before I allow you to send out any referrals," when the truth is medicare, or insurance will not pay the bills

one day past when the protocols say the patient is ready to move to skilled nursing.

➢ have to organize it when we are planning a family conference for all disciplines and 5 family members.

➢ get to sort out the complaints like, "this crisis was caused because of the hospital stay. It was your fault. Now you want to discharge my mom?!"

➢ know what to do when the patient asks, "What happens next? I don't understand any of this."

➢ help find the solution when the patient, clearly unable to manage alone at home, says, "None of my family can make me go to a nursing home! I am going home."

➢ are the ones the patient calls to say, "Neither the nurse nor the Home Health agency has called me since I left the hospital. You told me I would have a nurse at home."

➢ help the patient who says, "My doctor said I need to stay a few more days." when we know the insurance is denying further coverage starting today, and they have to let the doctor know that unless discharged the patient may get a bill, and the hospital will not get paid.

➤ know that although we incidentally found out that the patient has cancer, the insurance will only pay for what is necessary to stabilize this patient and the full work up has to continue after discharge, and are the ones to explain this to the doctors and the patient.

➤ despite all of the above, frequently hear, "Thank you for everything. We could not have done this without your help."

Patient Education

by Marianna Turgeon MSN RN CCM BSCS

Patient education and case management education go hand in hand. It is my experience that case managers are expected to have a solution to most, if not all issues regarding a patient discharge.

With a background as a labor and delivery nurse, I was not well versed in asthma or the administration of the appropriate medications for asthmatic patients. So, when I was charged with planning the discharge for a patient with asthma, I started researching.

I ran across a research article that stated that parents were surprisingly good about administering the asthma medications, but tended to forget about the maintenance and upkeep of the machine. The article stated there was a strong potentiality that they could inadvertently be reinfecting their children. The issue was that due to the small tubing diameter, even running water or a cleaning solution through it did not guarantee the tubing was clean.

I reached out to the respiratory therapist who worked for the medical equipment company and learned that the nebulizer tubing can be replaced several times a year. All the parent had to do was call the equipment provider (usually identifiable via a sticker on the side of the nebulizer) and ask for new tubing. Parents or patents could also ask for new tubing in their physician's office, because the offices usually kept replacement tubing and masks. The equipment supplier told me that when they deliver the nebulizers, they would discuss the cleaning instructions and reference the booklet provided with the nebulizer.

Once I learned this, I began providing this education to parents and patients as I planned their discharge home. Many parents thanked me for the education, because they said they had never been told about the maintenance of the nebulizers. Many said they would pass the information on to others.

Once during an assessment, I asked a grandfather who took care of his 10-year-old grandson who had cystic fibrosis, if his grandson had a nebulizer. I also inquired about how old it was and how often he used it. I explained that I learned parents were great about giving the medication, but sometimes forgot to clean the machine and mask. The grandfather looked at me with a "deer in the headlights" kind of look. He turned to his daughter and asked if this "cleaning and maintenance" pertained to continuous positive airway pressure (CPAP) machines too. The daughter looked at her father with the weirdest look and asked "Dad, why are you asking?" The grandfather said proudly, "Your mother used to take care of those things." His wife of 50 years passed about 5 years earlier from cancer and that is when he took on a major role of caring for his grandson.

His daughter said they did maintain her son's nebulizer, replacing the tubing and mask after every sickness. She also said she would look at her father's CPAP machine. She asked if we could possibly help with replacing accessories. I told her I could and would work with the grandfather's Pulmonologist or primary care physician to get him what he needed.

On the day of discharge, the daughter brought in her father's CPAP. She would not even handle it without gloves on. She put it in a clear, plastic bag and we could not believe what we saw. The whole inside length of the tubing had a black/gray haze. The daughter had taken the filters out of the CPAP the night before and they were a "charcoal" color instead of white as they were when new. She felt ashamed that her dad had been breathing through that mess for so many years, because he followed his doctor's instructions to use the CPAP every night.

I worked with the grandfather and we were able to get an appointment with his doctor in two days. We were also able to order a brand new CPAP that even turned out to be smaller and better than the old one. In addition, we were able to set him up with a new sleep study, because he had not had an appointment since his wife had passed. Case management has a wide range of impact and can support the whole family.

Who knew a case manager with a labor and delivery background would be able to provide important asthma education to families about the use of their asthma medication, the maintenance of their asthma machine and ensuring they had appropriate follow up appointments prior to discharge? And excitingly, I found my asthma education could extend to other members of the family.

The Lighthouse

by Eric Bergman RN BA CCM

Case management is the lighthouse in the night shining a path to protect patients from running aground in the dark.

Case management is the eye of the hurricane, where an overwhelmed and exhausted patient or family can breathe for a moment, focus, and get support for a plan to confidently re-enter the storm.

Case Management is air traffic control, coordinating the movement of many fast-moving and complex procedures, specialists, and organizations. The case manager guides everyone to coordinate the work, reconcile conflicts, and ensure everyone arrives safely at the end of the journey.

Case management is like a symphony orchestra conductor standing on a stage before a group of highly skilled professionals, each with a part to play in a complex performance, and guiding them all to work together while interpreting the work so that an audience (patients, families, insurance companies, government regulators, and communities) can absorb, understand and heal in the process.

Case managers spend their days sorting through complex issues that require a broad understanding of disease processes, treatments, and likely outcomes. Use their understanding of resources to support their clients. They must understand medical terminology and be able to communicate competently with specialists and medical professionals as well as translate the information into everyday language to communicate clearly with patients and families.

Our medical understanding and ability are expanding in wonderful ways every day, as we become ever more sophisticated and skilled at managing the amazingly complex machine that is the human body. However, that means that our treatments and medications are more difficult to understand and explain, and our systems can be mysterious to anyone without significant medical education, experience, and understanding. When people get seriously ill, they need support and guidance, and because many specialists must work together, that guidance requires specialization as well.

Case management is about interpretations, attention to detail, building relationships, and communicating clearly.

➢ We must interpret the medical events, terminology, results, and prognosis to ensure our patients and families understand what they are being told, so they can understand the choices they have to make, and the treatments they must endure.

➢ We must actively work to learn the details and ask the questions that elicit the answers doctors don't have time to explore or patients are reluctant to share. The little things often matter most.

➢ We must build relationships with patients to get the embarrassing or uncomfortable details that make all the difference between successful discharge and readmission, and that allow us to guide the medical team to coordinate and collaborate robustly when everyone is pressed for time.

➢ We must be able to explain the complex in simple terms and guide our patients to reliable information instead of the most popular trend on Dr. Google.

Case managers are the hub of the wheel that is complex medical care. Case management is the difference between mere treatment and a successful journey towards wellness.

Our Own Stories

"The stories we tell literally make the world. If you want to change the world, you need to change your story. This truth applies both to individuals and institutions." --Michael Margolis

My Journey

by Shawndel Pinnock, BSN, RN, CCM

Case management to me entails being a jack of all trades. Educator, liaison, coordinator, advocate, and a listening ear are some of the many titles a case manager could have, depending on one's area of specialty.

I first heard about case management as a brand-new floor nurse on a Medical-Surgical/Telemetry unit. My time as an overnight floor nurse was rough but was a wonderful learning experience for the short time I was there. Due to difficulty with work-life balance, I began searching for positions that would allow me to be available to my family at night and for the holidays. I applied to every job posting I could find, even positions that I may have not qualified for.

I finally got a call back from a company for a position as a Registered Nurse Care Coordinator. I thought to myself what could this entail, I only knew that it would involve working with children. It was finally time for the day of the interview. They had a clinic as well as multiple offices for different Nurse Care Coordinators. I interviewed well and was offered a position as a Nurse Care Coordinator.

Without fully understanding the position, I accepted because the timing was perfect for my family and me. Unbeknownst to me, this was the best decision I had ever made. I was able to have an impact on families without being physically involved like how I was in the hospital setting. I coordinated care by scheduling appointments, setting up transportation, identifying resources for families, and even sometimes helping parents obtain medications for their children.

Two years into my being a Nurse Care Coordinator, one of my colleagues suggested that I complete the certification to become a Certified Case Manager. I wasn't aware that there was a certification exam but I started doing research and was frightened by many people saying the exam was extremely hard. I later had to transition into another position due to company closure. I was once again with pediatrics but this time specializing in medical foster care and medically fragile children for a Managed Medical Assistance Program (MMA plan).

In my new position, I was considered interchangeably a Nurse Care Coordinator and a Concierge Nurse Care Coordinator. My members had many needs and had high acuity levels. I worked with each parent to the best of my ability to get the best outcome possible for each of the children that I was assigned to. I would always receive voicemails or calls from parents thanking me for my assistance, which made this job even more rewarding. One day once again with another coworker the CCM certification came up. I realized it was finally time for me to face my fears and look into becoming certified again.

I gave birth to my second child in March 2020 and one day while on maternity leave I decided enough is enough and I completed the application to get my certification. Not only did I want to achieve this goal for myself but I honestly could say that I love what I do and I love helping others behind the scenes. Many people take for granted their knowledge of certain benefits. During my time as a nurse care coordinator, I realized that there are a lot of people who could benefit from assistance and are unaware of the resources and people like myself who are available to help and advocate for them.

Fast forward to September 2020. I had many sleepless nights studying for a certification that I believed would further my knowledge and make me official. My testing day arrived and I am happy to say that I was able to pass this test. I know many may say this but I think I was destined to become a case manager especially by the mere fact of me landing my first position as a nurse care coordinator with no experience. It is now my passion to be able to advocate for others. Advocating for others has inadvertently helped me in my personal life. I was always the type of person that was scared to speak to people or even speak up for myself, but I now find myself advocating for not only myself but for my children and family as well. I now have a voice and I plan to continue to use it and help others as long as I can. I am excited to see what the future will bring on my path as a certified case manager. I plan to continue performing my many roles within case management and will continue to be an empathetic listener, a planner, a liaison, and a care coordinator to the best of my ability.

Making a Difference

by Victoria Chanda, CSW

I work as a Transitions of Care CM for a Medicaid MCO in Kentucky, the 46th poorest state in the US. To me, care management is helping a member who has been beaten by a boyfriend after having a stroke find stable, safe housing. It is helping an infant who was exposed to substances in utero and discharged to an ill-prepared family member get the support they need to make it a successful lasting placement. It is helping a gunshot victim piece their life back together in their newly traumatized and now physically impaired body. It is helping a homeless member connect to community resources that help them put food in their mouth and access medication.   It's helping a family get a handicap van so they can access the community in ways they have never been able to before.

Case management is also losses. It is logging into my computer in the morning and realizing the member who I helped get into rehab last week overdosed on heroin yesterday. It is relapses in pediatric cancer. It is denials of needed physical aids (DME). It is yet another change and another place to document. It is chasing down providers to get the prior authorization. It takes flexibility. A deep breath. And teamwork.

Case management is mobilizing during a pandemic to help members access the ever-changing processes in the health care world and helping them say goodbye to family members from a distance. It's bearing witness to their heartache.

Case management means being a jack of all trades; knowing payor sources, community resources, models of care, reimbursement structures, etc. It is knowing young and old, rural and urban. It is building relationships and networking with physicians, discharge planners, and DME companies. When working with people, the issues faced are as diverse as the members themselves.

Care management is celebrating the true successes like when a member achieves autonomy and meets their health goals.

It's busy, it's messy and at times overwhelming, it's documenting and then documenting it again.

It is getting up every day and helping problem-solve with the people that live in my community. It helps me count my blessings, make a difference, and know I am helping better the lives of those around me. COVID-19 has brought a lot of chaos to all of us, but being able to work from home and model nurturing, compassion, problem-solving, and grit to my children has been a blessing in disguise. It is knowing what I do matters and that at the end of the day, I have made a difference in my community.

When I Learned to Spell Case Management

by Mindy Owen, RN, CRRN, CCM

Thirty-seven years ago, my "nursing" career took a turn toward case management in Chicago. I was unsure what to expect. In fact, I could barely spell case management. Of the many lessons I have learned, one of the most important is to keep your eyes and mind wide open.

I became an RN in 1974 and, like many RNs, I began my career in a large acute medical center. We lived in Milwaukee, Wisconsin, so I applied and was hired by Milwaukee County Hospital, where my eyes were opened wide to all I did not know and needed to learn - quickly! Orientation was short, with the attitude "just get in and do it; if you need help, ask."

I was a staff nurse on a step-down ICU floor, grew into a Charge nurse for Neuro-ICU/ step-down, and gained a wealth of experience in 2 years. But then my husband's job moved us to Wichita, Kansas. We had never been there, or for that matter been that far from family, but we packed up for the adventure.

In Wichita, I looked for an ICU position, but there were none available . They asked if I would consider Neuro/Rehab (TBI/SCI). Initially I was disappointed, but thought I could do it until an ICU position was available. What I did not count on was that I would fall in love with Rehabilitation, the patients, and families we served. I became "Charge" and moved into the Director's position. I grew the program to CARF certification and, looking back, began to understand what made me "tick" as a healthcare professional.

I thrived on "planning", being an advocate for patients, families and staff, implementing programs and processes, facilitating a plan, and most of all, being part of a strong communication channel. Does any of that sound familiar in the practice of case management? I was asked to lead the start-up of the Kansas chapter of the Association of Rehabilitation Nurses (ARN), and 2 years later, I was elected to the National Board of ARN to serve as the Midwest Regional Director.

I led the Rehabilitation team at Wesley Medical Center in Wichita, Kansas for 8 years and would have continued, if we had not moved to Chicago. Chicago became home in 1984, and while we were excited, I was lost. I had thought my career would be as a Rehabilitation Nurse. However, in Chicago there were a couple of opportunities, but I felt they didn't fit me. Then a colleague suggested I go and speak with a company called Intracorp, a subsidiary of CIGNA.

I sent them a resume. When I met with the Director she told me "YOU would be a good case manager." I asked, "What's Case Management?" She said, "We're just beginning to explore that." However, she was sure I would be good at it?! I left her office confused, and went home to discuss the opportunity with my husband. I tried to find some information about case management, and quickly found it was extremely limited. Yet I decided to take a leap of faith. I learned that Intracorp and CIGNA had a vision and part of the vision was to develop and build a Case Management Model to serve acute healthcare patients with catastrophic injuries or illness and patients with chronic, long-term healthcare needs. Chicago was to be one of the anchors and while our team was small, we were dedicated and passionate to build a model reflective of case management for patients and families needing "coordinated continuity of care" and advocacy at their side. We worked hard, bridging the financial, clinical, therapeutic, and psycho-social aspects of healthcare. I became one of 13 members of the Case Management team nationwide that brought forward lessons learned and helped build the national model for Intracorp/Cigna case management.

It was during this time that several of us in Chicago, and around the country, were asked to explore organizing a national group to represent case management. An association management group in Washington D.C. named The Hill Group, organized a meeting of case management leaders from around the country, and I was included.

A group of about 12 people met at The Marriott near O'Hare airport in Chicago. We discussed the need for an organization to represent case management. The Hill Group indicated their willingness to assist us in developing a structure and helping to manage the organization, as well as subsidize the development. That day we decided on the name, The Case Management Society of America, (CMSA) We elected officers, and everyone wrote a check for $65.00 to launch the society.

We quickly realized that not only did we need to agree on a vision and mission, but would need to put voice to an agreed upon definition of case management. The Hill Group was based in Washington D.C. and guided us through our first public policy and lobbying efforts. They knew the timing was right to introduce case management into federal legislation. The definition was instrumental to beginning discussions related to the value of case management regarding healthcare legislation. Under their guidance we were able to have the definition of case management placed in the congressional record for the first time. It was a proud moment for CMSA.

As we enlisted colleagues and began to build a national organizational infrastructure, we believed strongly that it should be a chapter-driven society. Several of us in the Chicagoland area encouraged Chicago case managers to build a chapter. This was not easy. The Chicago group wanted to be independent, and they created The Illinois Case Management Network. It took several years before The Illinois CM Network would vote to become part of CMSA. Carrie Engen, now Carrie Marion, Nancy Skinner, Maureen Kretzer, and Tommie Lester, and other Chicago case management leaders were instrumental in launching The Illinois CM Network. I have always been grateful to have been part of the development of Case Management in Chicago, and nationally.

As we were building CMSA, both nationally and locally, certification was developing. The first certification commission for case management launched in Rolling Meadows, Illinois, a suburb of Chicago. This certification body had experience in certification of Rehabilitation Counselors, and Certified Disability Specialists. Case Management was a fit for them, but needed a structure to be built and validated. Several years after my term as the second National President of CMSA, I served on the CCM Commission for 11 years, chairing the commission twice.

Case managers have a unique skill set, one to be proud of, and to lean on that supports all the work we do. Chicago Case Managers are among the best, eager to learn, up for a challenge, and always ready with a hand extended to help a fellow case manager. I cherish my early days of case management in Chicago, where we were all learning together, recognizing differences and similarities in practice, building a model and process for those who would follow. Ultimately, we continue to build on the foundation I helped create many years ago.

In Closing

Case Managers are the key to creating a true patient centered care experience. Case Managers are an integral, but under used part of the healthcare team. Under used because the awareness of our existence is not wide enough yet.

For Our Patients and Their Families

Anyone who has any form of health insurance can access a case manager by calling the number on the back of their insurance care and "asking for a Case Manager." Case Managers are embedded in hospitals, clinics, community service agencies, and even practice independently in many communities. Every person deserves a Case Manager in their corner; we advocate, coordinate, and collaborate or the good of our patients and their families. If you need help finding a Case Manager, contact us at info@cmsa-chicago.org and "ask for a case manager." We will be happy to connect you with resources to find one.

For the Health Care Team

Just as Case Managers provide guidance and support for their patients/clients, one organization is providing more support, resources, forums, and outlets for the case management community than any other, Case Management Society of America (CMSA). Join us at www.cmsa.org

CMSA Chicago, is a local chapter of the Case Management Society of America (CMSA). It is the premier professional organization, providing education, networking and support to the entire case management community. CMSA Chicago brings everyone together to make navigating the health care system easier for the most important member of the health care team – the patient.

CMSA Chicago is here to support the entire case management community. Our scope of practice includes case managers in every setting across the continuum of care, as well as the myriad of service providers who offer a full spectrum of support to our mutual patients. We encourage you to attend an upcoming event and connect with your professional organization by visiting us at www.cmsa-chicago.org

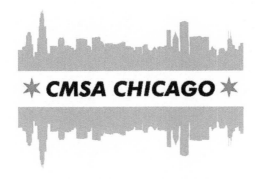

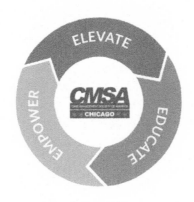

Made in the USA
Monee, IL
25 April 2021